THE PRIMAL BLUEPRINT

90-DAY
JOURNAL

n=1
A Personal Experiment

DISCLAIMER

The ideas, concepts and opinions expressed in this book are intended to be used for educational purposes only. This book is sold with the understanding that author and publisher are not rendering medical advice of any kind, nor is this book intended to replace medical advice, nor to diagnose, prescribe or treat any disease, condition, illness or injury. It is imperative that before beginning any diet or exercise program, including any aspect of the Primal Blueprint program, you receive full medical clearance from a licensed physician. Author and publisher claim no responsibility to any person or entity for any liability, loss, or damage caused or alleged to be caused directly or indirectly as a result of the use, application or interpretation of the material in this book. Sorry, but that's what my lawyers forced me to say in order for me to be able to offer you my insights. If you object to this disclaimer, you may return the book to the publisher for a full refund.

Library of Congress Control Number: 2012937984
Library of Congress Cataloging-in-Publication Data
Sisson, Mark, 1953–
The Primal Blueprint 90-Day Journal / Mark Sisson
ISBN: 9780984755141
1. Health 2. Weight Loss 3. Diet 4. Physical Fitness

Writing/Consulting: Brad Kearns
Design/Layout: Caroline DeVita
Editing/Research: Aaron Fox

For more information about The Primal Blueprint 90-Day Journal, please visit primalblueprint.com
For information on quantity discounts, please call 888-774-6259
Publisher: Primal Nutrition, Inc.
23805 Stuart Ranch Rd. Suite 145
Malibu, CA 90265

TABLE OF CONTENTS

BLOOD VALUES

RESOURCES

"Before, I had to eat every 2-3 hours or I would get lightheaded and even dizzy. Now I can do the odd 24-hour fast with no problem. I finally feel freed from my obsession with food, and the handcuffs of my eating timetable."

– Success Story Michelle

INTRODUCTION

As you might have gathered from a quick flip through the pages, *The Primal Blueprint 90-Day Journal - A Personal Experiment* aspires to transcend the overly structured, unimaginative – dare I say, lame – diet/exercise logs that populate bookstore shelves. This unique publication is designed to blend the best of both a practical and an intuitive approach – nurturing your creative, free-form expression while also serving as a scientific journal to gather empirical data about your personal experiments.

During my years as a competitive endurance athlete, I fastidiously logged my training – distances, times, routes – for years, but I'm not really sure why. Oh, I definitely took pleasure in filling those blanks with numbers; it celebrated and authenticated the hard work that I did out on the road. However, the hidden story behind the numbers was where the truly valuable insights were. What complementary lifestyle practices were in place when I was training at my best? Were there times when emotional disturbances (insecurity, impatience, frustration) negatively influenced my training decisions? Could patterns of overtraining leading to recurring injury and illness have been detected early on? Was I focused on the appreciation of the process, or getting too caught up in the numbers?

As a competitor, there is no escaping the reality that you have to do the requisite amount of work – put up the numbers – in order to become a champion. However, it is in the management of your distinct personality traits, emotions, and rational decision making that distinguishes the champion from the also ran. Effective journaling helps you identify and manage these intangible elements of peak performance – whether your goal is winning races, losing a few extra pounds, or creating more balance in your life. Journaling keeps you honest, focused and accountable to yourself. But you can't just go through the motions as you can with an ill-advised workout. You have to make a sincere effort to create a masterpiece within these pages for the next 90 days.

If you're a data wonk, go ahead and spit out all the details you want – wind speed during your sprints, barometric pressure during your pullups – whatever (there's plenty of room!). But I hereby challenge you to go deeper in this journal. Besides recording the facts, take advantage of the "open" format of this journal to relate how you feel – about meals, workouts, career and personal issues, and other lifestyle goals. Keep the thing under lock and key if you must, but don't hold anything back.

Blending the practical and the intuitive might feel a bit unfamiliar at first, particularly if you've become accustomed to the linear approach to pursuing goals favored by Conventional Wisdom. As you create your canvas over the next 90 days, take comfort in realizing that there is no right or wrong way to use this journal. Whatever works best for you is the best approach. You might leave entire sections blank for weeks on end if they don't resonate with you – no problem. Or you might expand upon minor elements of the journal pages and turn them into major ones.

The goal is to create a body of work that is meaningful and informative to you, and to gain a deeper appreciation for a process-oriented approach to setting and achieving goals. As they say, the numbers don't lie, but they are a little too reticent for my taste. Let the numbers fall where they may as you pursue a life of ease, contentment, enjoyment, and balance. If you have some OCD tendencies, see what happens when you loosen things up a little bit in your daily routine. If you're the type that has trouble getting motivated, write about what's in the way each day, take some baby steps when you feel overwhelmed, and revel in your progress, even if it's only inches at a time. Finally, remember that we're in this together: jump onto the MarksDailyApple.com Forum and visit the section devoted to Primal Blueprint Journals. You'll find lively commentary, helpful suggestions and general support for using this journal to its full advantage.

YOUR PERSONAL EXPERIMENT

$n=1$ is a scientific notation meaning literally, "a sample size of one". Over the next 90 days, you will hack and tweak numerous elements of your daily routine and record the results. We'll take a methodical approach here as follows:

STEP 1: Specify some **goals** you would like to accomplish over the next 90 days.

STEP 2: Design up to two **experiments** to help you achieve these goals, and track their progress over the next 90 days. Each experiment will state the goal ("lose weight; improve my 10k time; improve blood test results"), a hypothesis ("cutting carbs will result in weight loss; adding sprint workouts will improve my 10k time"), variables to introduce into your daily life, and measurements to track over time (See *How to Use: Personal Experiments* on pages 17-24).

STEP 3: Measure and record numerous **baseline values** relating to your health, daily routine, peak performance, and other measurements specific to your goals if they are not covered in the Baseline Evaluation.

STEP 4: Track progress. Use the blanks in the Experiment pages to make journal entries as desired. Re-measure baseline values at 30, 60, and 90 days and record in the Experiment pages.

If you haven't worn a lab coat or cracked a composition book in a while, I'll help you by providing some *n=1* examples with goals, hypotheses, variables, and measurements. You can conduct similar experiments, or take inspiration to design different experiments following the basic template.

Keep in mind that you're not trying to get a tenured professorship here; your approach will likely deviate from official scientific methods, and rightly so. For example, getting more sleep and conducting sprint workouts may both contribute to improved endurance performance. Attempting to somehow quantify these respective contributions would be impossible and also irrelevant. It's more important to think creatively, observe carefully how certain lifestyle practices improve, or compromise, your health, fitness, and quality of life, and learn from your *n=1* experiences to constantly grow and evolve. Record your data and track your variables carefully, but keep your eye on the big picture, and take guidance from this sign that hung in Albert Einstein's office: "Not everything that counts can be counted, and not everything that can be counted counts."

The Baseline Evaluation and Day 30, 60, and 90 Evaluations offer an opportunity to track your progress and quantify your results, both specific to your personal experiments and for general progress. As you can see, there are plenty of markers provided for you to measure, and dozens of additional custom options that you may choose to track, including some cool new stuff that can track fitness progress significantly better than the comparatively mundane tests favored by Conventional Wisdom.

BASELINE EVALUATION   3/5/12 DATE

DIET Past 90 days.

Energy	Dig M.	Health	Mood	Stress
6	8	8	7	4

Success Score: 6
Wins: Eating more from Farmer's Market
Challenges: Need to cut carbs in half! Not sure how family will adjust.

MACRONUTRIENT CALCULATIONS

Carbs	Protein	Fat	Calories
181	103	82	1,874

Comments: Looking forward to trying the online food journal. Will do immediate pantry cleanout, stop crappy snacks, start with Primal Essential Meals.

PRIMAL LIFESTYLE Past 90 days.

Success Score: 6

Sleep (1-10): 5   Comments: too much computer @ night. Stop @ 9pm - no exceptions!
Sun (1-10): N/A   Comments: Consider this after winter is over.
Play (1-10): 3   Comments: love the park play with the kids.
Brain (1-10): 7   Comments: Guitar lessons "totally count!" Ha!
Move (1-10): 3   Comments: Need to take regular breaks.

PERSONAL Past 90 days.

Comments: Need to have better balance between work and rest/workouts/ volunteering/kids

BASELINE EVALUATION

EXERCISE Past 90 days.

Success Score: 6   Effort score: 5
Wins: Good start with Primal Essential Movements.
Challenges: Hamstrings keep getting tight with sprints.
Comments: Try more easy wind sprints to get legs strong. Definitely make sure cardio sessions are 75% or less.

GOALS Goals/potential 90-day Personal Experiments.

1. Track average daily carb intake against body fat %
2. Calculate 06:03 ratios and reduce over 90 days.
3. Measure performance in PEMs and improve over 90 days.
4. _____
5. _____

BODY MEASUREMENTS

Time of Day: _____   Scale/method used: _____
Day 1 weight: 142 lbs   Day 1 fat %: _____
Day 2 weight: _____   Day 2 fat %: _____
Day 3 weight: _____   Day 3 fat %: _____
Average weight: _____   Average body fat %: _____

Body part measurements:.
Waistline: 28"   Hips: 35"   Chest: _____
Thighs: _____   Biceps: _____

Other body measurement: _____ Value: _____
Other body measurement: _____ Value: _____

Granted, it can be difficult and cost-prohibitive to run your blood or even test your body fat every 30 days. However, using online macronutrient calculators and conducting the

BASELINE EVALUATION

FITNESS MEASUREMENTS

Morning resting heart rate: __54__ __58__ __58__ Average: __56.6__
           Day 1   Day 2   Day 3

Maximum heart rate: __176__ Method: $208 - (.7 \times 46) = 176$
Aerobic exercise zone: __97__ to __132__
              55%   75%

Primal Essential Movements – one set maximum effort
Note type of progression or advanced exercise if not actual Essential Movement
(e.g. – decline pushups, chair-assisted pullups)
Pushups: __knee__ Number: __20__
Pullups: __chin up__ Number: __2__
Squats: __regular__ Number: __38__
Plank (time): __regular__ Time: __2:10__

400 meter run: _____ Date: _____
Location/conditions/notes: _____
One-mile run: __8:58__ Date: _____
Location/conditions/notes: __Venice Hi track, perfect weather.__
__Started out too fast! Can probably do an 8:30.__

Maximum Aerobic Function test
Date: __3/15/12__ Heart Rate: __130__
Course/distance: __Venice Hi track, 4 laps__ Time: __11:42__
Location/conditions/notes: _____
VO2 Max test (ml/kg value): _____
Date/location/method of test: _____

Other best performances:
Event/Exercise: __Circuit challenge at Mar Vista Park__ : Achievement: __6:23__
Event/Exercise: __3 laps w/ 5 pushups, 10 squats each ½-lap__ Achievement: _____
Event/Exercise: _____ Achievement: _____

fitness assessments described are free, and can reveal as much about health and fitness progress as an elaborate workup costing thousands of dollars at a medical/wellness spa. Be diligent about repeatedly testing the items of most importance to your health and fitness, particularly if you have medical issues.

DAILY JOURNAL ITEMS

1-10 Score grid: For your Baseline Evaluation, consider how things have gone over the past 90 days and give yourself a 1-10 Success Score. For the Day 30 and Day 60 Evaluations, score the previous 30-day periods. For your Day 90 Evaluation, score the entire 90-day journey.

"Big M": It's all about *Motivation* baby! Get your head around an intuitive approach to exercise, eating, and the pursuit of all peak performance goals. Sit quietly at the beginning of your day, prior to a workout, or prior to jumping into the fray at your office, and reflect on your daily motivation levels, along with other grid scores. Perhaps jot down a few notes in the Personal section about things that might be compromising a positive attitude and high motivation levels.

Health: General state of immune function; sore throat or stuffy head lowers score.

Stress: General level of daily stress and your success in managing it.

Macronutrients Calculations: Dialing in fat reduction is as simple as hitting the sweet spot on the Primal Blueprint Carbohydrate Curve with your average daily carb intake. While eating and living Primally is about flexibility, personal preference, and enjoyment of life, it may be helpful to occasionally track your macronutrient intake in a precise and methodical manner with an online food calculator. On the occasions that you generate reports online, fill in the blanks for carbs, protein, fat and total calories on those particular days. As you expand your knowledge of macronutrient values with help from online reports and the chart on page 279, you can input estimated figures on other days.

To obtain accurate values for your daily macronutrient intake, write down everything you eat, using measuring tools (cup with ¼ marks, tablespoon, ounces scale) to obtain quantities that are as accurate as possible. Carry around a small notepad so you don't forget anything. Visit Paleotrack.com and create a free account to begin entering data from your food journal (Fitday.com is another popular online journal). The Paleotrack interface is very simple and easy to learn: Just enter foods from your notes and a daily journal is generated. The journal displays a colorful pie chart representing macronutrient breakdowns, along with detailed calculations for amino acids, fatty acids, vitamins and minerals. Then, copy the data from Paleotrack into your 90-day journal; results will also be stored online in the Paleotrack database.

Most importantly, you must obtain adequate protein calories to preserve or build muscle tissue, and keep your carbohydrate intake in line with your body composition goals.

Average daily protein intake should be between .7 (minimally active) to 1 gram (highly active) of protein per pound of lean body mass per day. This is total bodyweight less fat weight; you can estimate this figure by guessing your body fat percentage and subtracting that amount of fat from your total weight. Carbohydrate intake goals are 50-100 grams per day for fat loss, and 100-150 to maintain ideal body composition. Keep in mind that these suggestions are averages, so try to journal your food intake during a normal day of eating. Or consider logging food intake for multiple days to get an accurate sense of your eating patterns.

The remaining calories that you obtain from fat should be just enough to make you feel totally satisfied at each meal or snack. As you become more and more fat- and keto-adapted from Primal eating/moderating insulin production, you will be better able to skip meals or otherwise moderate total daily fat intake to the extent that you obtain a significant portion of your daily energy requirements from storage depots on your body! Nailing your daily protein and carb requirements and optimizing your appetite and food intake patterns should enable a steady loss of between four and eight pounds of excess body fat per month. Consider the Primal Leap weight loss program at (visit **PrimalBlueprint.com** for details) if you require individualized support and guidance for your weight loss goals.

Generate an online report at least every 30 days to track your progress with Primal eating goals and enter the data into your evaluations pages. While the online data may be helpful if you are unfamiliar with macronutrient content of food, or struggling to progress at your goal pace, just cutting sugars and grains should default you into a weight maintenance zone or fat reduction zone.

Diet section: Summarize the most successful, and most challenging elements of your dietary habits over the past 90 days, as revealed in the sample journal on page 25.

Exercise section: Success Score refers to how well you feel your workouts have gone over the past 90 days. Have you achieved your fitness goals? Struggled with injuries, illness, or fluctuating motivation levels? Rate your success on 1-10 scale. Effort Score refers to how challenging your workout routine has been over the past 90 days.

Primal Lifestyle, Personal, and Goals sections are pretty straightforward. Reflect on the past 90 days, consider how things stand today, and list some of the major goals you would like to achieve during your 90-day personal experiment. We'll get into more detail with your goals in the Personal Experiments section.

BODY MEASUREMENTS

Weigh yourself at the same time of day with the same scale. Do it for three days in a row and take the average to allow for routine daily fluctuations in total bodyweight.

Body fat percentage can be measured easiest by skinfold calipers or a bioelectrical impedance scale. Proper use of calipers and bioelectrical impedance scales claim an accuracy rate of plus or minus three percent. Bioelectrical impedance scales (Tanita is the leading brand; decent models start around $50) run a microcurrent up through your bare feet standing on the scale and deliver an instant readout for total weight and body fat percentage.

Health clubs, universities and health professionals offer more sophisticated tests to produce (hopefully) greater accuracy, including underwater weighing, air displacement "pods", DEXA technology (which also measures muscle and bone density), and near-infrared spectroscopy. You can also just stand in front of a mirror, minimally clothed, and snap photos at regular intervals over time. Photos will clearly reveal even a couple percentage point changes in your body fat. Noticing how tight clothing fits will also reveal favorable improvements in body composition.

Body part measurements: If inclined, obtain some measurements with the help of a friend and a proper alteration measuring tape. Choose the widest part of your waist, hips, chest, thighs, and biceps while standing comfortably, with air exhaled. If you have any other measurements you wish to record, use the blanks in this section.

FITNESS MEASUREMENTS

Morning resting heart rate: Immediately upon awakening, make an effort to relax, count your pulse with a second hand for ten seconds and multiply by six. Resting heart rate is a reliable indicator of the stroke volume of your heart. A strong, fit heart will pump out more blood with each beat, and hence beat at a lower rate than someone who is unfit. Elite athletes commonly have resting heart rates in the forties, while an average resting heart rate is 72 beats per minute. See if you can lower yours over time as you improve your fitness.

Be alert for an elevated morning heart rate, which is a common sign of overtraining or general overstress. Anything 10 percent or more above the upper limit of your normal range warrants a reduction in exercise and life stress until resting heart rate returns to normal. For example, my normal, healthy resting heart rate ranges from 40-44 beats per minute. Recording a 48 or higher means I back off for a couple days.

Maximum heart rate: You can determine your maximum heart rate via a protocol for a strenuous lab or field test (get physician clearance) or estimate it using this formula: 208 minus (0.7 times age) = estimated maximum heart rate. For example, a 40-year-old has an estimated max heart rate of 180 beats per minute [208 - (.7 x 40) = 208 – 28 = 180].

Aerobic exercise zone: First, determine or estimate your maximum heart rate, then multiply that figure by 55 percent to determine the lower end of the zone, and 75 percent to determine the upper limit of the zone. Our 40-year-old example has an aerobic exercise zone of 99 beats (180 x .55) to 135 (180 x .75) beats per minute.

Make a point of frequently measuring your heart rate during exercise with a wireless heart rate monitor, or manually as follows: Get your heart working at a steady rhythm for a while, then stop and feel for the strong pulse emanating from the carotid artery on the side of your neck. Check your watch and count how many beats occur in exactly ten seconds. Multiply that number by six to determine your heart rate in beats per minute.

Seventy-five percent of max is surprisingly easy to exceed, since perceived effort at this intensity is moderate. Discipline and focus are required to stay in your target zone – even for experienced exercisers.

Primal Essential Movements: These exercises are described in detail in the Resources section. Please review the material and perform a Primal Essential Movements fitness assessment to determine your values for one set of maximum effort in each of the four exercises (specifying either progression, baseline or advanced exercise), as directed.

400-meter and One-mile run: These are excellent markers of cardiovascular fitness and even longevity. A 2011 study published by the University of Texas Southwestern Medical School and Cooper Institute in Dallas (of *Aerobics* fame) isolated the one-mile run time of a middle aged person as an excellent predictor of longevity and heart disease risk 30-40 years later as follows:

Males age 50+

- 8-minute mile: Excellent fitness
- 9-minute mile: Moderate fitness
- 10-minute+ mile: Low fitness

Females age 50+

- 9-minute mile: Excellent fitness
- 10:30-mile: Moderate fitness
- 12-minute+ mile: Low fitness

Excellent fitness level predicts a 10 percent lifetime risk of heart disease, while low fitness predicts a 30 percent lifetime risk of heart disease. Those with excellent fitness in their fifties are around twice as likely to reach age 85 as the unfit, and have eight years longer life expectancy than the unfit. Well, what are you waiting for? Get the stopwatch out and hit the track!

Maximum Aerobic Function (MAF) Test: This test measures your aerobic efficiency with a timed effort over a fixed course, at a fixed heart rate of 75 percent of your maximum. For example, running eight laps around a track while trying to keep your heart rate as close as possible to 130 beats per minute (or whatever your 75 percent figure is). A wireless heart rate monitor is required for accurate test results.

After a brief warmup, begin your test, taking care to get your heart rate quickly but smoothly up to 75 percent and then pegged there. Pay attention and alter your pace if your heart rate drifts higher or lower than your MAF test target number. Record your time for the eight laps (or other consistent course such as a specific hill climb on bicycle, a measured mile on road or trail, or going a certain distance on calibrated exercise equipment) and repeat the test every 30 days. Improving your time on a MAF test is a reliable indicator that you have become more efficient processing oxygen at low intensity. This is a great indicator of a general improvement in aerobic fitness, and correlates directly with being able to race faster at high intensity.

VO2 Max test: This test is typically conducted in a sports performance laboratory or advanced health, fitness or medical facility. It measures the volume of oxygen you can process at near maximum intensity, in relation to your bodyweight. Yep, strap an oxygen mask on your face and run on a treadmill till you collapse! Elite athletes have long used VO2 Max as a predictor of endurance potential. VO2 Max has far less "trainability" (able to improve score through training) than the MAF test, and is much more difficult and expensive to conduct. Focus on the MAF test and don't worry if you leave this one blank.

Other Best Performances: Perhaps you have some markers in your favorite sport or fitness activity you would like to record here? For the Baseline Evaluation, record your best achievement over the past 90 days, then repeat the test at 30, 60, and 90 days.

"BEFORE" AND "AFTER" PHOTOS

You may wish to establish a reference point by taking a full-body photograph while minimally clothed as part of your Baseline Evaluation. You can print the photo and affix it to a page provided at the end of the Baseline Evaluation. Room to affix another photo is provided as part of your Day 90 Evaluation. Who knows, maybe you'll submit them for the Success Stories section at MarksDailyApple.com!

How To Use: **PERSONAL EXPERIMENTS**

After completing the Baseline Evaluation, you will custom-design up to two experiments to conduct over the next 90 days. Start with the goals you mentioned in your Baseline Evaluation and pose a hypothesis for how you might succeed. For example, "Can I lose excess body fat by ditching grains and sugars from my diet?" Next, carefully consider the variables to introduce into your daily routine. Finally, specify the measurements you will track to evaluate results.

Create your personal experiments by pulling from the suggested experiments that follow, your general knowledge of the Primal philosophy, or another source of inspiration to try something that might work.

N=1 SAMPLE WORKSHEET

EXPERIMENT #1

Description: Drop 6lbs of fat and gain 2lbs of muscle in 45-60 days

Hypothesis: Follow Carb Curve + PEM workouts 2x/week to achieve goal

Variables:
1. Ditch grains and sugars
2. Do paleotrack.com report 1 day/week
3. Do PEM 2x/week plus aerobic + sprint workouts
4.
5.

Measurements:
1. Current fat % and total weight, repeat @ 30 days
2. Record PEM workouts - max effort assessment @ 30 days
3. Paleotrack reports 1 day/week - 100g or less carbs
4.
5.

Comments: Mom issues: Sweetened drinks (Lemonade), fresh mex (nacho quesadilla) → get bowls instead Go harder on PEMs but shorter sessions

EXPERIMENT #1

BASELINE MEASUREMENTS: Date: 2-4-12
Measurement: Weight   Value: 178lb
Measurement: Fat %   Value: 12.8% - Tanita
Measurement: Pushups   Value: 32
Measurement: Pullups   Value: 12
Measurement: Squats   Value: 63
            Planks   2:42
Comments: Wow great start on PEMs! Surprised at high total weight

30 DAY MEASUREMENTS: Date: March 6
Measurement: Weight   Value: 175lb
Measurement: Fat %   Value: 10.6% - Tanita
Measurement: Pushups   Value: 40
Measurement: Pullups   Value: 8 (elbow)
Measurement: Squats   Value: 64
            Planks   2:45
Comments: Feeling great and notice body comp changes. Try some I.F. next 30 days

60 DAY MEASUREMENTS: Date: April 10
Measurement: Weight   Value: 172lb
Measurement: Fat %   Value: 8.8 - Tanita
Measurement: Pushups   Value: 41

SAMPLE EXPERIMENT #1: REDUCE EXCESS BODY FAT

The hack here is to simply ditch grains, sugars and legumes from your diet and let results happen naturally. For a methodical approach, you can regularly track your carbohydrate intake with an online calculator, and follow the other suggestions listed to make your weight loss experience enjoyable and sustainable over the long run.

Hypothesis: Regulating carbohydrate intake into the range of 50-100 grams per day, combined with complementary Primal lifestyle practices, will enable a steady reduction of excess body fat.

Variables:

1. Moderate carb intake: Ditch grains, sugars and legumes and emphasize Primal foods. This should default you into the Carbohydrate Curve Sweet Spot without any sense of deprivation or struggle.

2. Track carb intake: Why take a chance that you won't succeed? Make a commitment to visit Paleotrack.com and log your daily food intake food intake for a day or two each week for the duration of your 90-day experiment. Evaluate the results and make adjustments to get your carb intake into the Sweet Spot if necessary.

3. Follow natural appetite: Eat when you are hungry, finish when satisfied. Eat all meals at a leisurely pace, in a calm, relaxed environment. Focus on the pleasure of eating delicious, Primal-approved foods. Reject negative influences such as guilt and rebellion from restrictive techniques and simply let your appetite guide your eating habits.

4. Try Intermittent Fasting: Strengthen your connection to hunger and satiety signals by occasionally (or frequently, as you become more Primal-aligned) skipping or delaying meals until you are actually hungry.

5. Exercise Primally: Eliminate Chronic Cardio patterns (which promote sugar cravings), increase all forms of daily movement (enhances fat burning) and conduct brief, high-intensity strength and sprint sessions (speeds metabolism, promotes lean muscle growth).

Measurements:

1. Record total body weight and body fat percentage at start, 30 days, 60 days and 90 days. Always measure in early morning using the same scale or measurement tools.

2. Use your daily journal to comment on Intermittent Fasting efforts and following natural appetite. Report a 1-10 score every 30 days for how well you are aligned with these dietary goals.

3. Use your daily journal to comment on your exercise habits, such as maintaining aerobic zone heart rates during sustained workouts, aligning workout effort scores with your 1-10 scores for daily energy, motivation, and health. Report a 1-10 score every 30 days for how well you adhere to the Primal exercise philosophy and eliminate Chronic Cardio patterns.

SAMPLE EXPERIMENT #2: IMPROVE ENDURANCE PERFORMANCE

Take a favorite event where you can easily repeat the performance: 5k run, one-mile run, bicycle time trial, competitive swimming event, a time/distance effort on a calibrated exercise machine, or your favorite 50-mile bike course or 15-mile trail run.

Hypothesis: Times can improve by adding high intensity workouts, increasing all forms of daily movement, and eliminating Chronic Cardio training patterns.

Variables:

1. Add one high-intensity sprint workout a week, following the protocol described on pages 266-267.

2. Find three ways to increase daily low-level movement. For example, walking at lunchtime or in the evening, taking stairs instead of elevators, or parking at the edge of parking lots.

3. Eliminate Chronic Cardio: Make a sincere effort to align workout degree of difficulty with your daily 1-10 scores for energy, motivation, and health. Maintain heart rate of 75 percent of maximum or less during sustained aerobic

workouts. Add 1-2 additional rest days and/or reduce overall workout volume if currently exceeding five hours per week of medium-to-difficult intensity (over 75 percent of max) sustained workouts.

Measurements:

1. Time chosen fitness event(s) at days 0, 30, 60 and 90. Attempt these timed performances only when feeling 100 percent energized and motivated, even if not exactly at specified checkpoint. Strive for identical weather conditions and other variables to preserve accuracy of results.

2. Track the 1-10 scores in your daily journal pages for the "Move" item in the Primal Lifestyle section. Report a 1-10 score every 30 days for how well you are aligned with daily movement.

3. Report a 1-10 score every 30 days for how well you adhere to the Primal exercise philosophy and eliminate Chronic Cardio patterns.

SAMPLE EXPERIMENT #3: IMPROVE BLOOD TEST RESULTS/REDUCE DISEASE RISK FACTORS

If you've been told by your doctor that you have some unfavorable blood numbers, or aren't sure where you stand and want to find out, test your blood at day 0 and again at day 90 of your experiment.

Hypothesis: Implementing Primal eating and lifestyle practices can improve assorted blood test values in under 30 days, with a virtual elimination of adverse values and disease risk factors in 90 days.

Variables:

1. Obtain starting values for as many items as possible on the Baseline Evaluation page (body weight, fat percentage, blood pressure, waistline, cholesterol, triglycerides, C-reactive protein, Lp2A, A1c and fasting blood glucose, fasting blood insulin, etc.)

2. Eliminate grains, sugars, and PUFA oils: Moderates insulin, lowers trigylcerides, raises HDL, reduces oxidation and inflammation.

3. Improve dietary omega-6:omega-3 (O6:O3) ratios: Reduces/protects against systemic inflammation. See next experiment for details.

4. Increase intake of saturated fat: Raises HDL, improves fat metabolism, regulates appetite.

5. Increase intake of antioxidants: Ditching grains and increasing intake of vegetables, fruits, nuts, seeds, herbs, spices and supplements will turbocharge antioxidant levels – your body's best natural defense against disease.

6. Exercise Primally (low level aerobic and brief, high intensity): raises HDL, lowers triglycerides and small, dense LDL.

Measurements:

1. Obtain blood tests at regular intervals from same laboratory, always in a fasted state or as otherwise directed by your doctor.

2. Report changes in other body measurements that may reveal improvements in disease risk factors, such as body weight, body fat percentage and body part measurements (as recorded in your Baseline, Day 30, Day 60 and Day 90 Evaluations).

SAMPLE EXPERIMENT #4: MODERATE SYSTEMIC INFLAMMATION

Systemic inflammation, believed to be the root cause of many common health problems and serious diseases, is triggered and exacerbated by overly stressful lifestyle practices (sleep deprivation, Chronic Cardio, hectic daily schedules) and poor dietary habits (excess carbohydrate intake, unfavorable omega-6:omega-3 ratios).

Hypothesis: Systemic inflammation can be moderated through diet and exercise modifications, resulting in an improvement of various aches, pains and specific health conditions (arthritis, tendonitis, colitis, etc.).

Variables:

1. Moderate carbohydrate intake/insulin production: Excessive glucose and insulin in the bloodstream is pro-inflammatory. Ditching grains, sugars and legumes in favor of Primal foods will moderate blood glucose and insulin levels.

2. Normalize O6:O3 ratios: Eliminate grains and PUFA oils, moderate intake of all nuts except macadamia, and increase intake of oily, cold water fish and omega-3 fish oil capsules.

3. Eliminate Chronic Cardio: Maintain heart rate of 75 percent of max or less during sustained aerobic workouts. Add 1-2 additional rest days and/or reduce overall workout volume if currently exceeding five hours per week of medium-to-difficult intensity sustained workouts.

4. Eliminate pain relief medication: Routine use of NSAIDs (aspirin, ibuprofen), Tylenol, or prescription corticosteroids or opioids can compromise your body's natural ability to moderate inflammation and mask pain that would otherwise limit activity to a sensible level. Try eliminating these meds for a period of time. This will allow your body's anti-inflammatory process to operate unimpeded, and natural sensations of pain to govern your activity. Combined with dietary modification, you may experience an improvement of inflammation-related conditions, particularly if you are patient and allow the experiment to run for 90 days.

Measurements:

1. Obtain blood tests at 0 and 90 days (or more frequently if desired), always in a fasted state or as otherwise directed by your doctor. Pay particular attention to the tests listed under "Inflammation Markers" in the instructions.

2. Track O6:O3 dietary ratio at regular intervals, inputting one or two days of food journals into Paleotrack.com and recording the O6:O3 ratios generated.

3. Rate the level of pain (1-10) in certain areas

4. Measure exercise performance(s) that you feel are directly affected/inhibited by systemic inflammation.

SAMPLE EXPERIMENT #5: IMPROVE SLEEPING HABITS

Assorted elements of modern life compromise optimal sleep habits, mainly artificial light and digital stimulation after dark, and overly stressful evening and morning rituals. These modern stressors interrupt natural hormone flows triggered by light and dark cycles, leading to assorted health problems.

Hypothesis: Aligning sleep habits more closely with my natural circadian rhythm will improve daily energy levels, exercise performance, fat reduction, and assorted health conditions. Better sleep means better performance in many other areas.

Variables:

1. Minimize artificial light and digital stimulation after dark: Consider using eyewear and light bulbs with a yellow or orange tint, particularly if you must interface with a screen after dark.

2. Implement calm, relaxing sleep rituals: Mellow out the final two hours before bed time, and sleep in a dark, cool, uncluttered room.

3. High-energy mornings: Awaken naturally, without an alarm clock, as close as possible to sunrise. If this is out of routine for you, exposure yourself to direct sunlight immediately upon awakening. This will train your body to awaken easier the next day.

Measurements:

1. Record in the daily journal a good estimate for the total hours of sleep you obtain each night. Calculate an average every 30 days and record on experiment page.

2. Report 1-10 score on overall quality of sleep over the past 90 days before beginning experiment. 10 would be a routine of deep, uninterrupted and restful sleep of at least eight hours each night, while a 1 would indicate chronic insomnia.

3. Report 1-10 score on morning energy levels/ease of awakening over the past 90 days: 10 for peppy early birds and 1 for pushing the snooze alarm multiple times.

4. Report 1-10 score on how mellow your evenings have been over the past 90 days:

10 would be evening strolls, quiet conversation and a good book by candlelight. 1 would be for Netflix doubleheaders taking you into the next calendar day before lights out.

5. Report 1-10 score for the aforementioned three categories at regular intervals during the experiment period. Ideally every two weeks but at least every 30 days. Refer to the 1-10 scores in your daily journal pages for the "Sleep" item in the Primal Lifestyle section for guidance.

"The best part about the Primal Blueprint is the freedom. Eat when you're hungry and stop when you're full. If you don't feel like exercising one day, don't worry about it."

– Success Story Deanna

DAY 1 WEEK 1   DATE: 4 / 1 / 12

1 - 10 SCORE

Energy	Big M.*	Health	Mood	Stress
7	7	9	9	1

DATA

Weight	Fat %	Foot	Knee
161	7.7	2	0

MACRONUTRIENT CALCULATIONS

Carbs	Protein	Fat	Calories
112	122	165	2,335

DIET Success Score: 7

Meals: 10:15am - Primal smoothie (2 scoop, ½ banana, ½ can coco milk, flakes, ice) = Perfect!
2:3pm - Tuna salad stuffed red pepper (pesto + sundried tomato)
7pm - Thompson Wagyu ground beef w/ Mozarella, onions, peppers, squash
Snacks: Mac nuts, carrots in pm. Dark chocolate (Ethereal from Santa Barbara waters) at Farhad's art show
Comments: Whole Foods run - coco milk, flakes, salsa, beets kale, red cabbage. Diestel turkeys - ordered 2 for par. Morning energy fine so 14hr fast

PRIMAL LIFESTYLE Success Score: 8

Sleep (1-10): 8   Comments: Lites out 10:20pm Woke 6:30am
Sun (1-10): N/A   Comments: Cloudy April
Play (1-10): 7   Comments: Frisbee dogs 5pm
Brain (1-10): 6   Comments: A few drum lesson drills pm
Move (1-10): 7   Comments: Gettin dogs out 2x/day = 3 great

PERSONAL

Comments: Email discipline going okay. Try 1 hour start in am Then block out period

EXERCISE Success Score: 8   Effort Score: 8

Workout: "Skyridge 100"   Duration: 20 min
Location: Skyridge Loop
Exercise 1: Decline pushups Weight: ___ Reps/Time: 30 Set 2: ___ Set 3: ___
Exercise 2: Decline - trail Weight: ___ Reps/Time: 25 Set 2: ___ Set 3: ___
Exercise 3: Decline - wall Weight: ___ Reps/Time: 15 Set 2: ___ Set 3: ___
Exercise 4: Decline - picnic Weight: ___ Reps/Time: 8 Set 2: ___ Set 3: ___
Exercise 5: Decline - upper lot Weight: ___ Reps/Time: 20 Set 2: ___ Set 3: ___
Exercise 6: Decline - dugout Weight: ___ Reps/Time: 12 Set 2: ___ Set 3: ___
Comments: 110!
Sprints: 2x grass, 2x upper field, 1x uphill drive
Jog 5 min before and after. Elbow fine

Workout: Frisbee Dogs   Distance: ___   Duration: 15 min
Location: 5pm RaThead
Comments: 60x Spiderman, 60x Frog Squat // Jog/walk 15 m.

SUMMARY

Tomorrow: Bball 11:45am - warmup fully
This Week: Love PEM Isolation. Try pullups / frog squats combo
This Month: Track 400m trial next
Wins: Love PEM Isolation. Try pullups / frog squats combo
Challenges: Do n=1 for morning meal time / I.F
Comments: More frog squats - help knee

One Word: Nice! I like!   Success Score (1-10): 10

There are 90 days of Daily Journal (two-page) spreads, color-coded into 13 different weeks. You will date each day of the journal manually, allowing you to begin whenever you like and proceed for 90 days. You may prefer to begin your journal on a Monday, in order to have the familiar five-day workweek and two-day weekend in the same numbered week section. Ideally, you will deliver 90 consecutive days of journaling, but you may decide to put the log aside for a certain period time if major life disruptions occur (illness, lengthy business trip, crazy holiday schedule, etc.), and resume devoted journaling efforts when things get back to normal.

A quick glance at a daily two-page spread reveals a ton of opportunity to record data. Don't be overwhelmed! Remember, it's perfectly acceptable to skip sections that don't apply, or make brief comments in large sections. Mainly, I want to make sure that you have all the space you need in the major areas. Each day, the categories to comment on are your 1-10 Score grid, Data grid, Macronutrient calculations (from online data or estimate), Diet details, Primal Lifestyle elements, specific Personal issues you are facing, Exercise details, and Summary information. Following is an overview of each of the categories and other elements of the daily spread and how to best use them.

COLORED DATE HEADING

Manually enter the date each day. Numbering each week is mainly for your convenience; let's not make too big a deal of it. Think of a bigger picture, such as the 30, 60 and 90-day checkpoints that you will journal about. Realize that while workweeks and weekends are an important structural element of modern society, a week represents an arbitrary block of time to your body. The process of fitness, weight loss, and health happens dynamically and is in constant fluctuation. Many people make the mistake of fixating on weekly mileage, weekly weight loss or the like, and consequently overtrain or become discouraged just because a seven-day period did not go perfectly as planned.

"1-10 SCORE" GRID

Fill in a subjective score for each of these lifestyle elements as described on page 10-11. Complete the grid at the same time of the day for consistency. I like to track these items upon waking; others might prefer to complete the grid at the end of a busy day. Ideally, you'd slap down eights and tens into this grid each day. However, when you start noticing a downward trend with these numbers over a few days or even weeks, you will be able to identify lifestyle variables that are compromising your scores and take corrective action.

DATA GRID

If you are the type that likes to weigh yourself frequently – hey, there's a box for you. Fat % = body fat percentage, using a bioelectrical impedance scale or calipers. Once a week entry is plenty here. The blank boxes x1 and x2 allow you to custom-track quantifiable data from personal experiments of all kinds, both health-related and otherwise. Be creative…or, leave them blank – it's up to you! Some examples:

- 1-10 score on injuries/health problems (knee, plantar fascitis, carpal tunnel, etc.)
- Time tracking: Minutes spent reading with child, training dog, or meeting with co-workers
- Inclusion/exclusion variables in your daily routine: Foods, stretching, workout particulars, sleep/wake times, morning or evening rituals
- Medical data: Blood pressure, fasting blood glucose, morning body temperature, or other readings that you like to take daily, or at least more frequently than the Evaluations every 30 days

Some of these items may also be chronicled in detail in the Personal Experiments section, located just before Daily Journal spreads, at intervals of your choosing.

MACRONUTRIENT CALCULATIONS

Refer to the detailed instructions for generating data from online food journal in the Evaluation pages instructions. You can also use this grid to estimate your daily macronutrient intake, with assistance from the chart on page 279 at the back of the journal.

DIET SECTION

Assess an overall success score for the day's food choices and meal satisfaction. Meal and snack comments can include what you ate in as much detail as you wish. Under comments, you may want to list where and what you shopped for or a certain recipe that you prepared. Also feel free to detail any positive or negative emotional elements about your eating, or how you enjoyed meals in general.

PRIMAL LIFESTYLE SECTION

Give yourself a 1-10 rating for how well you honored the various Primal Blueprint lifestyle law categories each day. While details are discussed in *The Primal Blueprint*, here are some brief reminders of what you are looking for:

Sleep: Did you align your sleep habits with circadian rhythm, winding things down after sunset with calm, relaxing evenings of minimal digital stimulation and artificial light? Did you awaken close to sunrise, refreshed and energized, without requiring an alarm clock? This would result in a 9 or 10 score. I don't think I need to describe what a 1 or 2 score looks like here!

Sun: During the peak months of solar intensity in your location, did you expose large skin surface areas of your body to sufficient sunlight to facilitate vitamin D production? The rule of thumb is to stay in the sun for about half the time it would take to sustain a sunburn. Maintaining a slight tan, in season, indicates healthy vitamin D levels.

Remember, the key is large skin surface areas, so don't be shy about exposing. If you have fair skin or are otherwise concerned about overexposure in sensitive areas such as face and neck, go ahead and screen them routinely. They don't contribute much toward vitamin D production anyway. If you are using the log in wintertime when vitamin D production is impossible at your latitude, this entry will have minimal relevance, although you can comment when consuming vitamin D supplements.

Play: We're looking for regular efforts to take even brief breaks during your busy day for some spontaneous, outdoor physical fun. Did you have time to fetch the ball or Frisbee with the dog? Hit the jungle gym with the kids? Play hacky sack with co-workers in the office courtyard? Throw a few 10's onto the chart when you enjoy major weekend outings for new adventures!

Brain: "Use Your Brain" involves creative intellectual pursuits that balance the grind of your core daily responsibilities: Crosswords, Sudoku, Zynga games, brain teasers, memorizing song lyrics, adding numbers in your head. Put up some 10's if you venture out to take music lessons or complete a foreign language course.

Move: Look for creative ways to increase general everyday movement. Pay particular attention to breaking up long sedentary periods with even a brief five-minute stroll or quick jaunt up and down the office stairwell. Establish some habits such as parking at the edge of parking lots, eschewing elevators, and taking a quick neighborhood stroll after dinner before winding down for the evening. Put up some 10's if you bicycle to the weekend farmer's market or walk that mile to and from the commuter train station.

PERSONAL SECTION

I purposely left the Personal section open-ended, or shall we say, personal?! You don't even need to title the topic you are writing about! This is where you can riff on those communication issues with your teenager, the state of office politics, relationship drama, or anything else of a personal nature that comes to mind each day. If you have ongoing "issues" such as the aforementioned, you may even wish to use the x1 and x2 grid boxes to establish daily 1-10 scores for these matters, and elaborate with comments in this section.

EXERCISE SECTION

Each day, sections for two different types of workouts are provided. The first workout section is designed for a strength training, interval or other session consisting of multiple exercises, with data fields for weight, reps/time and a second or third set of the same exercise. The second workout section has less detail, making it suitable for aerobic sessions, hikes, sprint workouts, play sessions, or competitive games begging for more free-form commentary.

The Success Score and Effort Score blanks at the beginning of the section are critical. Please take the time to carefully evaluate the Success Score of your workout, relative to how you enjoyed it, whether you accomplished what you planned to, and how your mind and body responded to the effort. The Effort Score is simply a 1-10 value for how difficult the workout was. The goal here is to notice a trend of these 1-10 scores aligning closely with the figures in the 1-10 Score Grid (Energy, Motivation, Health, etc.).

SUMMARY SECTION

Tomorrow, This Week, and This Month allow you to comment on short-term goals that you aspire to. For the most part, you'll want to reference upcoming big workouts, food journaling days, or play sessions, but it's okay to record other stuff unrelated to health and fitness goals if they're on your mind. For example, packing or running errands for an imminent vacation.

Wins and Challenges relate to the general feelings you have about the issues of the day. These are designed to be brief answers about items you perhaps already answered in the journal ("Wins: great PEM workout; Primal meals; good day at work"). Take a few moments to prepare some summary comments for each day, along with a single word (or two…) and number on a 1-10 scale that best captures your overall feeling about the day.

How To Use: **BLOOD VALUES**

Following are many health-critical items to measure from blood tests or by other methods. Tracking blood work is a highly specialized and individualized wellness endeavor, and you may wish to consult with a medical doctor or alternative health care professional to determine items of most interest and importance to you. While being outside generally accepted normal ranges with your test results is something definitely worth paying attention to and engaging in further discussion, remember that all lab work is a snapshot of one moment in time and that values can fluctuate from day to day.

If you are not inclined to submit to a blood test or have medical insurance limitations on what you can order up without paying exorbitant fees, don't worry about leaving this section blank. However, if you test your blood regularly or are dealing with disease risk factors currently, consider consulting with your physician and/or laboratory about ordering some of these less common tests that can reveal important information about your health. For example, your triglycerides-to-HDL ratio is more relevant to heart disease risk than the commonly touted total LDL measurement. Testing for high sensitivity C-reactive protein (something that might not be a included in a routine blood panel) can indicate systemic inflammation and related health problems that are brewing without immediate symptoms.

BLOOD CHEMISTRY

Blood Pressure: High blood pressure (hypertension) is a major public health threat and one of the leading causes of death in the USA. Hypertension puts excessive stress on the cardiovascular system, increasing the risk of heart attacks, strokes, aneurysms, and kidney failure. It is caused by unhealthy lifestyle practices, such as excessive intake of carbohydrates, sodium (largely from processed foods), and PUFA fats, poor sleep habits, insufficient exercise, smoking, high levels of life stress, and genetic factors. Most medical experts believe the safe blood pressure threshold is a diastolic/systolic reading of 120/80 or lower (for each number).

Complete Blood Count (CBC): The bread and butter of blood tests, your CBC reveals an assortment of values with accepted normal ranges for each value.

Hematocrit (Hct; or PCV – packed cell volume): Measures the percentage of your blood that is comprised of red blood cells. Normal level for males is 45 (45%); 40 for females. Healthy levels facilitate efficient oxygen transport. This is of particular interest to endurance athletes and the reason why doping to increase hematocrit is a common practice. Low hematocrit levels can indicate anemia or overtraining, although athletic training has a tendency to slightly lower hematocrit naturally (perhaps due to increased blood volume diluting red blood cell percentage). Dehydration can result in a temporary elevation of hematocrit due to blood becoming more concentrated.

Iron: A critical component of blood health and oxygen processing. There are various lab tests associated with your levels of iron in the bloodstream as well as in storage, including serum iron, TIBC, serum ferritin and percentage of iron saturation. Talk to your health care provider if you believe you are at risk of iron deficiency (growing youth, hard training female athletes, Chronic Cardio enthusiasts).

White blood cells (leukocytes): Immune cells that defend the body against infectious disease. Elevated levels can indicate the presence of disease.

Vitamin D: A critical health marker often overlooked by mainstream practitioners and routine blood panels. Adequate vitamin D levels support optimal hormone function and healthy cell division (and thus prevention of all forms of cancer, including melanoma). Be sure to obtain the most relevant test for the circulating form of vitamin D in the bloodstream, called "25-vitamin D" or "serum 25(OH)D". Test in early fall for peak levels after a summer of (hopefully) adequate sun exposure. Diet contributes insignificantly to your requirements; it's all about getting enough sun during the season, and taking supplements if necessary.

Vitamin D expert Dr. Michael Holick (author of *The Vitamin D Solution*) recommends maintaining a range of 40-60 ng/ml, and believes that anything under 30 is deficient. Vitamin D deficiency is a serious public health problem affecting millions of modern citizens, but has no overt symptoms. If you have uncertainty about your sun exposure, or have skin pigment incongruent with your latitude (e.g. of African descent living in Sweden), get checked! Home tests are available from zrtlab.com for $75.

Fasting blood insulin: High fasting insulin levels are indicative of prediabetic conditions – residual evidence of the routine excessive overproduction of insulin.

HbA1C (estimated average glucose): Measures how much glucose is attached to a hemoglobin molecule, a reliable marker for the dangers of elevated blood glucose levels over an extended time period. This is a superior test to the more common instantaneous blood glucose readings (something commonly tracked by diabetics with a portable machine) that vary throughout the day and are strongly influenced by meals.

Plasma viscosity: High values correlate with athletic performance; low values correlate with overtraining.

Glutamine: Amino acid critical to healthy immune function and cellular repair. Low values can indicate overtraining.

Other values: Note other values of importance from your panel, particularly those that fell outside the average range. Consider obtaining a complete urinalysis for other valuable data. Females: ask for beta HCG on your urinalysis if you menstruate.

INFLAMMATION MARKERS

High sensitivity–C-reactive protein (hs-CRP): The medical community sets a "low risk" CRP threshold at 1.0mg/L or less. In the absence of other acute infections, high levels of hs-CRP in your blood are associated with an increased risk of heart attack, stroke, and sudden cardiac death. "Normal" CRP levels are supposedly 10 mg/L. Absent infection or acute stressors, however, ideal CRP levels are well under 1 mg/L. Between 10-40 mg/L (and perhaps even 1-9 mg/L, too) indicates systemic inflammation (or pregnancy), while anything above that is associated with a serious acute condition (e.g., heart attack, major infection, post-marathon or Ironman race).

IL-6, or Interleukin-6: T cells (type of white blood cell that plays a huge role in the immune response) and macrophages (cells that engulf and digest – also known as phagocytosing – stray tissue and pathogens) both secrete IL-6 as part of the inflammatory response, so elevated IL-6 can indicate systemic inflammation.

Lp2A: Another key inflammation marker associated with small, dense LDL particles.

Homocysteine: An amino acid that when elevated can increase risk of heart attacks, strokes, and blood clots. Vitamin and mineral deficiences can lead to elevated levels too, making it a good general health marker to track.

Creatine phosphokinase (CPK): Enzyme found in brain and lungs (CPK-1) heart (CPK-2), and skeletal muscle (CPK-3). Elevated levels indicate damaged tissues, from a medical incident or extreme athletic stress.

Omega-6/3 serum test: An excess of omega-6 in relation to omega-3 can promote systemic inflammation. Unfavorable ratios are typical of the Standard American Diet (SAD), and can even be a problem when eating Primally. You can also track O6:O3 ratios by food journaling at Paleotrack.com. A pattern of excessive dietary O6:O3 ratios predicts poor blood results. Experts believe that an ideal ratio is 2:1 or better, while SAD eating delivers ratios of 20:1 or even worse!

Omega-3 bodily tissue content: Omega-3 and omega-6 both convert into eicosanoids in the body. These are anti-inflammatory (O3) or pro-inflammatory (O6) signaling molecules. An omega-3 content of around 60 percent is ideal. An excess of omega-6 will promote systemic inflammation.

Omega-3 index: Measures EPA and DHA, the two important omega-3 fatty acids, as a percentage of total fatty acids present in your red blood cells. If you have a low omega-3 index, you are probably sporting excessive omega-6 in your red blood cells. Experts suggest that 12-15 percent is ideal. Above eight percent is "low risk". Four percent and below is "high risk" for systemic inflammation.

Other tests for inflammation or autoimmune disorders: EBV panel, ANA panel, complete cytokine assay, candida antibodies, helicobacter IgG panel, Hep A, B and C titers, breakout of cytokine panel, ESR, RA factor, SLE screen, T Lymphocyte helper suppressor assay, IL 8, IL 1 B or TNF alpha analysis.

LIPIDS

Readers of *The Primal Blueprint* will be familiar with my discussion of LDL particle size in association with heart disease risk. Briefly, small, dense LDL particles can be problematic, while large, fluffy LDLs are generally harmless. Furthermore, one's general state of oxidation and inflammation in the bloodstream represents the true catalyst for heart disease; obsessing on LDL values foolishly oversimplifies the issue. The following tests can shed valuable additional insights about your lipid risk factors.

Apolipoprotein B (ApoB): Measures a protein residing in all LDL particles. High levels indicate elevated heart disease risk. Request this test with your physician and discuss your readings in the context of normal ranges. Keep in mind that ApoB readings can fluctuate from day to day and provide only a snapshot of the health status of your cardiovascular system over time.

Triglyceride:HDL ratio: Experts such as Dr. Catherine Shanahan, author of *Deep Nutrition* and *Food Rules*, tout this test as a premier marker for heart disease risk, or lack thereof. A ratio of 3.5:1 or less is recommended, with 1:1 or better being outstanding. A favorable ratio indicates that you have a preponderance of large, fluffy LDL, as well as plenty of HDL to scavenge the bloodstream for potentially damaging agents.

Total Cholesterol: Mostly meaningless without further context. Nevertheless, compiling all the possible figures will provide clues to your heart health.

HDL (High-density lipoprotein): Popular reading for "good" cholesterol. HDL scavenges the bloodstream, removing waste products, returning LDL cholesterol to the liver for recycling, and helping keep artery walls clean and healthy. High HDL values are believed to reduce risk of heart disease, with experts recommending a level above 60 for excellent protection.

LDL (Low-density lipoprotein): Popular reading for "bad" cholesterol, although large, fluffy particles are harmless and only small, dense particles should be of any concern. Worth measuring over the long run, since numbers trending higher can indicate poor LDL clearance from blood (and greater chance of oxidation and potential damage). Offers better context when particle sizes and sub-fractions are identified.

Triglycerides: Exceeding 150 mg/dl indicates more oxidized LDL and thus poor health and elevated heart disease risk. Strive to get triglycerides below 100 mg/dl.

Total Cholesterol-to-HDL ratio: Calculating your total cholesterol to HDL ratio can help provide further context to your lipid values. Lower is better.

HORMONES

Testosterone: Predominant male hormone promoting strength, power, endurance, recovery, and even cognitive function. Also critical to female health in smaller amounts. Test for total testosterone, free testosterone, and percentage of free testosterone.

Cortisol: Elevated levels can indicate excess life stress, while low levels can indicate burnout. Test for both serum and salivary levels.

Thyroid: Numerous values are tested; best to order a complete panel with antibody screening.

Melatonin: Can indicate the quality of your sleeping habits as insufficient sleep can result in low melatonin levels.

Other Hormones: DHT, LH, FSH, Estradiol (E2) high sensitivity, DHEA-S (precursor to sex hormones), IGF-1 (insulin growth factor). Home testing kits for many hormones are available from zrtlabs.com.

CANCER SCREENINGS

Talk to your physician about your risk factors and the most appropriate cancer screenings to obtain. Some of the common tests are CEA for colon, CA 125 for ovarian, CA 27.29 for breast, and PSA for prostate (although this test has come under scrutiny recently for being unreliable).

SUBJECTIVE EVALUATIONS

- **Autoimmune flare-ups:** Sore joints, dry/patchy/red skin, mild arthritis.
- **Stress reactions or mannerisms:** Chewing your nails, pulling your hair out, etc.
- **Persistent nasal congestion:** Can also be due to food or environmental allergies, but even these are triggered by inflammation.
- **Overtraining:** Lack of typical energy/endurance/explosive strength, sore joints and muscles, irritable mood, poor immune function.

BASELINE EVALUATION

/ / DATE

DIET Past 90 days.

Success Score:_____

Wins:_____

Challenges:_____

Comments:_____

_____

_____

_____

_____

1 - 10 SCORE

Energy:	"Big M":	Health:	Mood:	Stress:

MACRONUTRIENT CALCULATIONS

Carbs:	Protein:	Fat:	Calories:

PRIMAL LIFESTYLE Past 90 days.

Success Score:_____

Sleep (1-10):_____   Comments:_____

Sun (1-10):_____   Comments:_____

Play (1-10):_____   Comments:_____

Brain (1-10):_____   Comments:_____

Move (1-10):_____   Comments:_____

PERSONAL Past 90 days.

Comments:_____

_____

_____

_____

_____

_____

_____

_____

BASELINE EVALUATION

EXERCISE   Past 90 days.

Success Score:_____   Effort Score:_____

Wins:_____

Challenges:_____

Comments:_____

_____

_____

_____

GOALS   Goals/potential 90-day Personal Experiments.

1._____

2._____

3._____

4._____

5._____

BODY MEASUREMENTS

Time of Day:_____   Scale/method used:_____

Day 1 weight:_____   Day 1 fat %:_____

Day 2 weight:_____   Day 2 fat %:_____

Day 3 weight:_____   Day 3 fat %:_____

Average weight:_____   Average body fat %:_____

Body part measurements:.

Waistline:_____ Hips:_____ Chest:_____

Thighs:_____ Biceps:_____

Other body measurement:_____ Value:_____

Other body measurement:_____ Value:_____

BASELINE EVALUATION

FITNESS MEASUREMENTS

Morning resting heart rate:_____ _____ _____ Average:_____
                                Day 1   Day 2   Day 3

Maximum heart rate:_____ Method:_____

Aerobic exercise zone:_____ to _____
                            55%   75%

Primal Essential Movements – one set maximum effort

Note type of progression or advanced exercise if not actual Essential Movement
(e.g. – decline pushups, chair-assisted pullups)

Pushups:_____ Number:_____

Pullups:_____ Number:_____

Squats:_____ Number:_____

Plank:_____ Time:_____

400-meter run:_____ Date:_____

Location/conditions/notes:_____

One-mile run:_____ Date:_____

Location/conditions/notes:_____
_____

Maximum Aerobic Function test

Date:_____ Heart Rate:_____

Course/distance:_____ Time:_____

Location/conditions/notes:_____

VO2 Max test (ml/kg value):_____

Date/location/method of test:_____

Other best performances:

Event/Exercise:_____ Achievement:_____

Event/Exercise:_____ Achievement:_____

Event/Exercise:_____ Achievement:_____

Affix "Before" photo here.

Comments on "Before" photo:_____
_____
_____
_____

EXPERIMENT #1

Description:_____
_____
_____
_____

Hypothesis:_____
_____
_____

Variables:

1._____
2._____
3._____
4._____
5._____

Measurements:

1._____
2._____
3._____
4._____
5._____

Comments:_____
_____
_____
_____
_____

EXPERIMENT #1

BASELINE MEASUREMENTS: Date:_____

Measurement:_____ Value:_____

Measurement:_____ Value:_____

Measurement:_____ Value:_____

Measurement:_____ Value:_____

Measurement:_____ Value:_____

Comments:_____

_____

_____

_____

DAY 30 MEASUREMENTS: Date:_____

Measurement:_____ Value:_____

Measurement:_____ Value:_____

Measurement:_____ Value:_____

Measurement:_____ Value:_____

Measurement:_____ Value:_____

Comments:_____

_____

_____

_____

DAY 60 MEASUREMENTS: Date:_____

Measurement:_____ Value:_____

Measurement:_____ Value:_____

Measurement:_____ Value:_____

EXPERIMENT #1

Measurement:_____ Value:_____

Measurement:_____ Value:_____

Comments:_____

_____

_____

_____

_____

DAY 90 MEASUREMENTS: Date:_____

Measurement:_____ Value:_____

Measurement:_____ Value:_____

Measurement:_____ Value:_____

Measurement:_____ Value:_____

Measurement:_____ Value:_____

Comments:_____

_____

_____

_____

_____

OBSERVATIONS/COMMENTS:

Date:_____

Comments:_____

_____

_____

_____

_____

EXPERIMENT #1

Date:_____

Comments:_____

_____

_____

_____

_____

Date:_____

Comments:_____

_____

_____

_____

_____

Date:_____

Comments:_____

_____

_____

_____

_____

Date:_____

Comments:_____

_____

_____

_____

_____

EXPERIMENT #2

Description:_____

_____

_____

_____

Hypothesis:_____

_____

_____

Variables:

1._____
2._____
3._____
4._____
5._____

Measurements:

1._____
2._____
3._____
4._____
5._____

Comments:_____

_____

_____

_____

_____

EXPERIMENT #2

BASELINE MEASUREMENTS: Date:_____

Measurement:_____ Value:_____

Measurement:_____ Value:_____

Measurement:_____ Value:_____

Measurement:_____ Value:_____

Measurement:_____ Value:_____

Comments:_____

_____

_____

_____

DAY 30 MEASUREMENTS: Date:_____

Measurement:_____ Value:_____

Measurement:_____ Value:_____

Measurement:_____ Value:_____

Measurement:_____ Value:_____

Measurement:_____ Value:_____

Comments:_____

_____

_____

_____

DAY 60 MEASUREMENTS: Date:_____

Measurement:_____ Value:_____

Measurement:_____ Value:_____

Measurement:_____ Value:_____

EXPERIMENT #2

Measurement:_____ Value:_____

Measurement:_____ Value:_____

Comments:_____

_____

_____

_____

_____

DAY 90 MEASUREMENTS: Date:_____

Measurement:_____ Value:_____

Measurement:_____ Value:_____

Measurement:_____ Value:_____

Measurement:_____ Value:_____

Measurement:_____ Value:_____

Comments:_____

_____

_____

_____

_____

OBSERVATIONS/COMMENTS:

Date:_____

Comments:_____

_____

_____

_____

_____

EXPERIMENT #2

Date:_____
Comments:_____
_____
_____
_____
_____

Date:_____
Comments:_____
_____
_____
_____
_____

Date:_____
Comments:_____
_____
_____
_____
_____

Date:_____
Comments:_____
_____
_____
_____
_____

DAY 1
WEEK 1

DATE / /

1 - 10 SCORE

Energy:	"Big M":	Health:	Mood:	Stress:

DIET   Success Score:_____

Meals:_____

_____

_____

_____

_____

DATA

Weight:	Fat %:	x1:_____	x2:_____

MACRONUTRIENT CALCULATIONS

Carbs:	Protein:	Fat:	Calories:

_____

_____

_____

_____

_____

Snacks:_____

_____

Comments:_____

_____

_____

_____

PRIMAL LIFESTYLE   Success Score:_____

Sleep (1-10):_____   Comments:_____

Sun (1-10):_____   Comments:_____

Play (1-10):_____   Comments:_____

Brain (1-10):_____   Comments:_____

Move (1-10):_____   Comments:_____

PERSONAL

Comments:_____

_____

_____

_____

EXERCISE

Success Score:_____ Effort Score:_____

Workout:_____

Location:_____ Duration:_____

Exercise 1:_____ Weight:_____ Reps/Time:_____ Set 2:_____ Set 3:_____

Exercise 2:_____ Weight:_____ Reps/Time:_____ Set 2:_____ Set 3:_____

Exercise 3:_____ Weight:_____ Reps/Time:_____ Set 2:_____ Set 3:_____

Exercise 4:_____ Weight:_____ Reps/Time:_____ Set 2:_____ Set 3:_____

Exercise 5:_____ Weight:_____ Reps/Time:_____ Set 2:_____ Set 3:_____

Exercise 6:_____ Weight:_____ Reps/Time:_____ Set 2:_____ Set 3:_____

Comments:_____
_____
_____
_____
_____

Workout:_____

Location:_____ Distance:_____ Duration:_____

Comments:_____
_____
_____
_____

SUMMARY

Tomorrow:_____

This Week:_____ This Month:_____

Wins:_____

Challenges:_____

Comments:_____
_____
_____
_____
_____

One Word   Success Score (1-10)

DAY 2
WEEK 1

DATE
/ /

Energy:	"Big M":	Health:	Mood:	Stress:

DIET
Success Score:_____

Meals:_____

_____

_____

_____

_____

DATA

Weight:	Fat %:	$x1$: _____	$x2$: _____

MACRONUTRIENT CALCULATIONS

Carbs:	Protein:	Fat:	Calories:

_____

_____

_____

_____

Snacks:_____

_____

Comments:_____

_____

_____

_____

PRIMAL LIFESTYLE
Success Score:_____

Sleep (1-10):_____ Comments:_____
Sun (1-10):_____ Comments:_____
Play (1-10):_____ Comments:_____
Brain (1-10):_____ Comments:_____
Move (1-10):_____ Comments:_____

PERSONAL

Comments:_____

_____

_____

_____

EXERCISE   Success Score:_____   Effort Score:_____

Workout:_____

Location:_____ Duration:_____

Exercise 1:_____ Weight:_____ Reps/Time:_____ Set 2:_____ Set 3:_____

Exercise 2:_____ Weight:_____ Reps/Time:_____ Set 2:_____ Set 3:_____

Exercise 3:_____ Weight:_____ Reps/Time:_____ Set 2:_____ Set 3:_____

Exercise 4:_____ Weight:_____ Reps/Time:_____ Set 2:_____ Set 3:_____

Exercise 5:_____ Weight:_____ Reps/Time:_____ Set 2:_____ Set 3:_____

Exercise 6:_____ Weight:_____ Reps/Time:_____ Set 2:_____ Set 3:_____

Comments:_____

_____

_____

_____

_____

Workout:_____

Location:_____ Distance:_____ Duration:_____

Comments:_____

_____

_____

_____

_____

SUMMARY

Tomorrow:_____

This Week:_____ This Month:_____

Wins:_____

Challenges:_____

Comments:_____

_____

_____

_____

_____

_____

One Word   Success Score (1-10)

DAY 3
WEEK 1

DATE / /

1 - 10 SCORE

Energy:	"Big M":	Health:	Mood:	Stress:

DIET

Success Score:_____

Meals:_____

_____

_____

_____

_____

DATA

Weight:	Fat %:	x1: _____	x2: _____

MACRONUTRIENT CALCULATIONS

Carbs:	Protein:	Fat:	Calories:

_____

_____

_____

_____

Snacks:_____

_____

Comments:_____

_____

_____

_____

PRIMAL LIFESTYLE

Success Score:_____

Sleep (1-10):_____ Comments:_____

Sun (1-10):_____ Comments:_____

Play (1-10):_____ Comments:_____

Brain (1-10):_____ Comments:_____

Move (1-10):_____ Comments:_____

PERSONAL

Comments:_____

_____

_____

_____

EXERCISE   Success Score:_____   Effort Score:_____

Workout:_____

Location:_____ Duration:_____

Exercise 1:_____ Weight:_____ Reps/Time:_____ Set 2:_____ Set 3:_____

Exercise 2:_____ Weight:_____ Reps/Time:_____ Set 2:_____ Set 3:_____

Exercise 3:_____ Weight:_____ Reps/Time:_____ Set 2:_____ Set 3:_____

Exercise 4:_____ Weight:_____ Reps/Time:_____ Set 2:_____ Set 3:_____

Exercise 5:_____ Weight:_____ Reps/Time:_____ Set 2:_____ Set 3:_____

Exercise 6:_____ Weight:_____ Reps/Time:_____ Set 2:_____ Set 3:_____

Comments:_____

_____

_____

_____

_____

Workout:_____

Location:_____ Distance:_____ Duration:_____

Comments:_____

_____

_____

_____

_____

SUMMARY

Tomorrow:_____

This Week:_____ This Month:_____

Wins:_____

Challenges:_____

Comments:_____

_____

_____

_____   _____

_____

                                    One Word   Success Score (1-10)

DAY 4
WEEK 1

DATE
/ /

1 - 10 SCORE

Energy:	"Big M":	Health:	Mood:	Stress:

DIET

Success Score:_____

Meals:_____

_____

_____

_____

DATA

Weight:	Fat %:	x1: _____	x2: _____

MACRONUTRIENT CALCULATIONS

Carbs:	Protein:	Fat:	Calories:

_____

_____

_____

_____

Snacks:_____

_____

Comments:_____

_____

_____

_____

PRIMAL LIFESTYLE

Success Score:_____

Sleep (1-10):_____   Comments:_____
Sun (1-10):_____   Comments:_____
Play (1-10):_____   Comments:_____
Brain (1-10):_____   Comments:_____
Move (1-10):_____   Comments:_____

PERSONAL

Comments:_____

_____

_____

_____

EXERCISE Success Score:_____ Effort Score:_____

Workout:_____

Location:_____ Duration:_____

Exercise 1:_____ Weight:_____ Reps/Time:_____ Set 2:_____ Set 3:_____

Exercise 2:_____ Weight:_____ Reps/Time:_____ Set 2:_____ Set 3:_____

Exercise 3:_____ Weight:_____ Reps/Time:_____ Set 2:_____ Set 3:_____

Exercise 4:_____ Weight:_____ Reps/Time:_____ Set 2:_____ Set 3:_____

Exercise 5:_____ Weight:_____ Reps/Time:_____ Set 2:_____ Set 3:_____

Exercise 6:_____ Weight:_____ Reps/Time:_____ Set 2:_____ Set 3:_____

Comments:_____

_____

_____

_____

_____

Workout:_____

Location:_____ Distance:_____ Duration:_____

Comments:_____

_____

_____

_____

SUMMARY

Tomorrow:_____

This Week:_____ This Month:_____

Wins:_____

Challenges:_____

Comments:_____

_____

_____

_____

_____

One Word   Success Score (1-10)

DAY 5
WEEK 1

DATE

/ /

1 - 10 SCORE

Energy:	"Big M":	Health:	Mood:	Stress:

DIET

Success Score:_____

Meals:_____

_____

_____

_____

_____

_____

_____

_____

_____

Snacks:_____

Comments:_____

_____

_____

_____

DATA

Weight:	Fat %:	x1: _____	x2: _____

MACRONUTRIENT CALCULATIONS

Carbs:	Protein:	Fat:	Calories:

PRIMAL LIFESTYLE

Success Score:_____

Sleep (1-10):_____ Comments:_____

Sun (1-10):_____ Comments:_____

Play (1-10):_____ Comments:_____

Brain (1-10):_____ Comments:_____

Move (1-10):_____ Comments:_____

PERSONAL

Comments:_____

_____

_____

_____

EXERCISE Success Score:_____ Effort Score:_____

Workout:_____

Location:_____ Duration:_____

Exercise 1:_____ Weight:_____ Reps/Time:_____ Set 2:_____ Set 3:_____

Exercise 2:_____ Weight:_____ Reps/Time:_____ Set 2:_____ Set 3:_____

Exercise 3:_____ Weight:_____ Reps/Time:_____ Set 2:_____ Set 3:_____

Exercise 4:_____ Weight:_____ Reps/Time:_____ Set 2:_____ Set 3:_____

Exercise 5:_____ Weight:_____ Reps/Time:_____ Set 2:_____ Set 3:_____

Exercise 6:_____ Weight:_____ Reps/Time:_____ Set 2:_____ Set 3:_____

Comments:_____

_____

_____

_____

_____

Workout:_____

Location:_____ Distance:_____ Duration:_____

Comments:_____

_____

_____

_____

SUMMARY

Tomorrow:_____

This Week:_____ This Month:_____

Wins:_____

Challenges:_____

Comments:_____

_____

_____

_____

_____

_____

One Word   Success Score (1-10)

DAY 6
WEEK 1

DATE __/__/__

1 - 10 SCORE

Energy:	"Big M":	Health:	Mood:	Stress:

DIET

Success Score:_____

Meals:_____
_____
_____
_____
_____

DATA

Weight:	Fat %:	x1: _____	x2: _____

MACRONUTRIENT CALCULATIONS

Carbs:	Protein:	Fat:	Calories:

_____
_____
_____
_____
_____

Snacks:_____
_____

Comments:_____
_____
_____
_____

PRIMAL LIFESTYLE

Success Score:_____

Sleep (1-10):_____   Comments:_____
Sun (1-10):_____   Comments:_____
Play (1-10):_____   Comments:_____
Brain (1-10):_____   Comments:_____
Move (1-10):_____   Comments:_____

PERSONAL

Comments:_____
_____
_____
_____

EXERCISE   Success Score:_____   Effort Score:_____

Workout:_____

Location:_____ Duration:_____

Exercise 1:_____ Weight:_____ Reps/Time:_____ Set 2:_____ Set 3:_____

Exercise 2:_____ Weight:_____ Reps/Time:_____ Set 2:_____ Set 3:_____

Exercise 3:_____ Weight:_____ Reps/Time:_____ Set 2:_____ Set 3:_____

Exercise 4:_____ Weight:_____ Reps/Time:_____ Set 2:_____ Set 3:_____

Exercise 5:_____ Weight:_____ Reps/Time:_____ Set 2:_____ Set 3:_____

Exercise 6:_____ Weight:_____ Reps/Time:_____ Set 2:_____ Set 3:_____

Comments:_____

_____

_____

_____

_____

Workout:_____

Location:_____ Distance:_____ Duration:_____

Comments:_____

_____

_____

_____

SUMMARY

Tomorrow:_____

This Week:_____ This Month:_____

Wins:_____

Challenges:_____

Comments:_____

_____

_____

_____

_____

_____

One Word   Success Score (1-10)

DAY 7
WEEK 1

DATE __ / __ / __

Energy:	"Big M":	Health:	Mood:	Stress:

DIET

Success Score:_____

Meals:_____

_____

DATA

Weight:	Fat %:	x1: _____	x2: _____

MACRONUTRIENT CALCULATIONS

Carbs:	Protein:	Fat:	Calories:

_____

_____

_____

_____

_____

Snacks:_____

Comments:_____

_____

_____

_____

PRIMAL LIFESTYLE

Success Score:_____

Sleep (1-10):_____   Comments:_____

Sun (1-10):_____   Comments:_____

Play (1-10):_____   Comments:_____

Brain (1-10):_____   Comments:_____

Move (1-10):_____   Comments:_____

PERSONAL

Comments:_____

_____

_____

_____

EXERCISE

Success Score:_____ Effort Score:_____

Workout:_____

Location:_____ Duration:_____

Exercise 1:_____Weight:_____Reps/Time:_____Set 2:_____Set 3:_____

Exercise 2:_____Weight:_____Reps/Time:_____Set 2:_____Set 3:_____

Exercise 3:_____Weight:_____Reps/Time:_____Set 2:_____Set 3:_____

Exercise 4:_____Weight:_____Reps/Time:_____Set 2:_____Set 3:_____

Exercise 5:_____Weight:_____Reps/Time:_____Set 2:_____Set 3:_____

Exercise 6:_____Weight:_____Reps/Time:_____Set 2:_____Set 3:_____

Comments:_____

_____

_____

_____

_____

Workout:_____

Location:_____ Distance:_____ Duration:_____

Comments:_____

_____

_____

_____

SUMMARY

Tomorrow:_____

This Week:_____ This Month:_____

Wins:_____

Challenges:_____

Comments:_____

_____

_____

_____

_____

One Word

Success Score (1-10)

DAY 8
WEEK 2

DATE
/ /

1 - 10 SCORE

Energy:	"Big M":	Health:	Mood:	Stress:

DIET   Success Score:_____

Meals:_____

_____

_____

_____

_____

DATA

Weight:	Fat %:	x1: _____	x2: _____

MACRONUTRIENT CALCULATIONS

Carbs:	Protein:	Fat:	Calories:

_____

_____

_____

_____

Snacks:_____

_____

Comments:_____

_____

_____

_____

PRIMAL LIFESTYLE   Success Score:_____

Sleep (1-10):_____   Comments:_____

Sun (1-10):_____   Comments:_____

Play (1-10):_____   Comments:_____

Brain (1-10):_____   Comments:_____

Move (1-10):_____   Comments:_____

PERSONAL

Comments:_____

_____

_____

_____

EXERCISE   Success Score:_____   Effort Score:_____

Workout:_____

Location:_____ Duration:_____

Exercise 1:_____ Weight:_____ Reps/Time:_____ Set 2:_____ Set 3:_____

Exercise 2:_____ Weight:_____ Reps/Time:_____ Set 2:_____ Set 3:_____

Exercise 3:_____ Weight:_____ Reps/Time:_____ Set 2:_____ Set 3:_____

Exercise 4:_____ Weight:_____ Reps/Time:_____ Set 2:_____ Set 3:_____

Exercise 5:_____ Weight:_____ Reps/Time:_____ Set 2:_____ Set 3:_____

Exercise 6:_____ Weight:_____ Reps/Time:_____ Set 2:_____ Set 3:_____

Comments:_____

_____

_____

_____

_____

Workout:_____

Location:_____ Distance:_____ Duration:_____

Comments:_____

_____

_____

_____

_____

SUMMARY

Tomorrow:_____

This Week:_____ This Month:_____

Wins:_____

Challenges:_____

Comments:_____

_____

_____

_____

_____

_____

One Word   Success Score (1-10)

DAY 9
WEEK 2

DATE ___/___/___

1 - 10 SCORE

Energy:	"Big M":	Health:	Mood:	Stress:

DIET

Success Score:_____

Meals:_____

_____

_____

_____

_____

DATA

Weight:	Fat %:	x1: _____	x2: _____

MACRONUTRIENT CALCULATIONS

Carbs:	Protein:	Fat:	Calories:

_____

_____

_____

_____

Snacks:_____

_____

Comments:_____

_____

_____

_____

PRIMAL LIFESTYLE

Success Score:_____

Sleep (1-10):_____ Comments:_____

Sun (1-10):_____ Comments:_____

Play (1-10):_____ Comments:_____

Brain (1-10):_____ Comments:_____

Move (1-10):_____ Comments:_____

PERSONAL

Comments:_____

_____

_____

_____

EXERCISE   Success Score:_____   Effort Score:_____

Workout:_____

Location:_____ Duration:_____

Exercise 1:_____ Weight:_____ Reps/Time:_____ Set 2:_____ Set 3:_____

Exercise 2:_____ Weight:_____ Reps/Time:_____ Set 2:_____ Set 3:_____

Exercise 3:_____ Weight:_____ Reps/Time:_____ Set 2:_____ Set 3:_____

Exercise 4:_____ Weight:_____ Reps/Time:_____ Set 2:_____ Set 3:_____

Exercise 5:_____ Weight:_____ Reps/Time:_____ Set 2:_____ Set 3:_____

Exercise 6:_____ Weight:_____ Reps/Time:_____ Set 2:_____ Set 3:_____

Comments:_____

_____

_____

_____

_____

Workout:_____

Location:_____ Distance:_____ Duration:_____

Comments:_____

_____

_____

_____

SUMMARY

Tomorrow:_____

This Week:_____ This Month:_____

Wins:_____

Challenges:_____

Comments:_____

_____

_____

_____

_____ | One Word | Success Score (1-10) |

_____

One Word   Success Score (1-10)

DAY 10
WEEK 2

DATE / /

1 - 10 SCORE

Energy:	"Big M":	Health:	Mood:	Stress:

DIET Success Score:_____

DATA

Weight:	Fat %:	x1: _____	x2: _____

Meals:_____

MACRONUTRIENT CALCULATIONS

Carbs:	Protein:	Fat:	Calories:

_____

_____

_____

_____

_____

_____

_____

_____

Snacks:_____

_____

Comments:_____

_____

_____

_____

PRIMAL LIFESTYLE Success Score:_____

Sleep (1-10):_____ Comments:_____

Sun (1-10):_____ Comments:_____

Play (1-10):_____ Comments:_____

Brain (1-10):_____ Comments:_____

Move (1-10):_____ Comments:_____

PERSONAL

Comments:_____

_____

_____

_____

EXERCISE

Success Score:_____ Effort Score:_____

Workout:_____

Location:_____ Duration:_____

Exercise 1:_____ Weight:_____ Reps/Time:_____ Set 2:_____ Set 3:_____

Exercise 2:_____ Weight:_____ Reps/Time:_____ Set 2:_____ Set 3:_____

Exercise 3:_____ Weight:_____ Reps/Time:_____ Set 2:_____ Set 3:_____

Exercise 4:_____ Weight:_____ Reps/Time:_____ Set 2:_____ Set 3:_____

Exercise 5:_____ Weight:_____ Reps/Time:_____ Set 2:_____ Set 3:_____

Exercise 6:_____ Weight:_____ Reps/Time:_____ Set 2:_____ Set 3:_____

Comments:_____

_____

_____

_____

_____

Workout:_____

Location:_____ Distance:_____ Duration:_____

Comments:_____

_____

_____

_____

SUMMARY

Tomorrow:_____

This Week:_____ This Month:_____

Wins:_____

Challenges:_____

Comments:_____

_____

_____

_____

_____

_____

One Word

Success Score (1-10)

DAY 11
WEEK 2

DATE / /

DIET   Success Score:_____

Meals:_____

_____

_____

_____

DATA

Weight:	Fat %:	x1: _____	x2: _____

MACRONUTRIENT CALCULATIONS

Carbs:	Protein:	Fat:	Calories:

_____

_____

_____

_____

Snacks:_____

_____

Comments:_____

_____

_____

_____

PRIMAL LIFESTYLE   Success Score:_____

Sleep (1-10):_____   Comments:_____
Sun (1-10):_____   Comments:_____
Play (1-10):_____   Comments:_____
Brain (1-10):_____   Comments:_____
Move (1-10):_____   Comments:_____

PERSONAL

Comments:_____

_____

_____

_____

EXERCISE   Success Score:_____   Effort Score:_____

Workout:_____

Location:_____ Duration:_____

Exercise 1:_____ Weight:_____ Reps/Time:_____ Set 2:_____ Set 3:_____

Exercise 2:_____ Weight:_____ Reps/Time:_____ Set 2:_____ Set 3:_____

Exercise 3:_____ Weight:_____ Reps/Time:_____ Set 2:_____ Set 3:_____

Exercise 4:_____ Weight:_____ Reps/Time:_____ Set 2:_____ Set 3:_____

Exercise 5:_____ Weight:_____ Reps/Time:_____ Set 2:_____ Set 3:_____

Exercise 6:_____ Weight:_____ Reps/Time:_____ Set 2:_____ Set 3:_____

Comments:_____
_____
_____
_____
_____

Workout:_____

Location:_____ Distance:_____ Duration:_____

Comments:_____
_____
_____
_____
_____

SUMMARY

Tomorrow:_____

This Week:_____ This Month:_____

Wins:_____

Challenges:_____

Comments:_____
_____
_____
_____
_____

One Word	Success Score (1-10)

DAY 12

WEEK 2

1 - 10 SCORE

Energy:	"Big M":	Health:	Mood:	Stress:

DIET

Success Score:_____

Meals:_____

_____

_____

_____

DATA

Weight:	Fat %:	x1: _____	x2: _____

MACRONUTRIENT CALCULATIONS

Carbs:	Protein:	Fat:	Calories:

_____

_____

_____

_____

_____

Snacks:_____

_____

Comments:_____

_____

_____

_____

PRIMAL LIFESTYLE

Success Score:_____

Sleep (1-10):_____ Comments:_____

Sun (1-10):_____ Comments:_____

Play (1-10):_____ Comments:_____

Brain (1-10):_____ Comments:_____

Move (1-10):_____ Comments:_____

PERSONAL

Comments:_____

_____

_____

_____

EXERCISE   Success Score:_____   Effort Score:_____

Workout:_____

Location:_____   Duration:_____

Exercise 1:_____	Weight:_____	Reps/Time:_____	Set 2:_____	Set 3:_____
Exercise 2:_____	Weight:_____	Reps/Time:_____	Set 2:_____	Set 3:_____
Exercise 3:_____	Weight:_____	Reps/Time:_____	Set 2:_____	Set 3:_____
Exercise 4:_____	Weight:_____	Reps/Time:_____	Set 2:_____	Set 3:_____
Exercise 5:_____	Weight:_____	Reps/Time:_____	Set 2:_____	Set 3:_____
Exercise 6:_____	Weight:_____	Reps/Time:_____	Set 2:_____	Set 3:_____

Comments:_____

_____

_____

_____

_____

Workout:_____

Location:_____   Distance:_____   Duration:_____

Comments:_____

_____

_____

_____

_____

SUMMARY

Tomorrow:_____

This Week:_____   This Month:_____

Wins:_____

Challenges:_____

Comments:_____

_____

_____

_____

_____

| One Word | Success Score (1-10) |

DAY 13
WEEK 2

DATE / /

1 - 10 SCORE

Energy:	"Big M":	Health:	Mood:	Stress:

DIET

Success Score:_____

Meals:_____

_____

DATA

Weight:	Fat %:	x1: _____	x2: _____

MACRONUTRIENT CALCULATIONS

Carbs:	Protein:	Fat:	Calories:

_____

_____

_____

_____

_____

_____

Snacks:_____

_____

Comments:_____

_____

_____

_____

PRIMAL LIFESTYLE

Success Score:_____

Sleep (1-10):_____ Comments:_____

Sun (1-10):_____ Comments:_____

Play (1-10):_____ Comments:_____

Brain (1-10):_____ Comments:_____

Move (1-10):_____ Comments:_____

PERSONAL

Comments:_____

_____

_____

_____

EXERCISE   Success Score:_____   Effort Score:_____

Workout:_____

Location:_____ Duration:_____

Exercise 1:_____ Weight:_____ Reps/Time:_____ Set 2:_____ Set 3:_____

Exercise 2:_____ Weight:_____ Reps/Time:_____ Set 2:_____ Set 3:_____

Exercise 3:_____ Weight:_____ Reps/Time:_____ Set 2:_____ Set 3:_____

Exercise 4:_____ Weight:_____ Reps/Time:_____ Set 2:_____ Set 3:_____

Exercise 5:_____ Weight:_____ Reps/Time:_____ Set 2:_____ Set 3:_____

Exercise 6:_____ Weight:_____ Reps/Time:_____ Set 2:_____ Set 3:_____

Comments:_____

_____

_____

_____

_____

Workout:_____

Location:_____ Distance:_____ Duration:_____

Comments:_____

_____

_____

_____

SUMMARY

Tomorrow:_____

This Week:_____ This Month:_____

Wins:_____

Challenges:_____

Comments:_____

_____

_____

_____

_____

One Word	Success Score (1-10)

DAY 14
WEEK 2

DATE / /

1 - 10 SCORE

Energy:	"Big M":	Health:	Mood:	Stress:

DIET   Success Score:_____

Meals:_____

_____

_____

_____

DATA

Weight:	Fat %:	x1: _____	x2: _____

MACRONUTRIENT CALCULATIONS

Carbs:	Protein:	Fat:	Calories:

_____

_____

_____

_____

Snacks:_____

_____

Comments:_____

_____

_____

_____

PRIMAL LIFESTYLE   Success Score:_____

Sleep (1-10):_____ Comments:_____

Sun (1-10):_____ Comments:_____

Play (1-10):_____ Comments:_____

Brain (1-10):_____ Comments:_____

Move (1-10):_____ Comments:_____

PERSONAL

Comments:_____

_____

_____

_____

EXERCISE

Success Score:_____   Effort Score:_____

Workout:_____

Location:_____ Duration:_____

Exercise 1:_____ Weight:_____ Reps/Time:_____ Set 2:_____ Set 3:_____

Exercise 2:_____ Weight:_____ Reps/Time:_____ Set 2:_____ Set 3:_____

Exercise 3:_____ Weight:_____ Reps/Time:_____ Set 2:_____ Set 3:_____

Exercise 4:_____ Weight:_____ Reps/Time:_____ Set 2:_____ Set 3:_____

Exercise 5:_____ Weight:_____ Reps/Time:_____ Set 2:_____ Set 3:_____

Exercise 6:_____ Weight:_____ Reps/Time:_____ Set 2:_____ Set 3:_____

Comments:_____

_____

_____

_____

_____

Workout:_____

Location:_____ Distance:_____ Duration:_____

Comments:_____

_____

_____

_____

_____

SUMMARY

Tomorrow:_____

This Week:_____ This Month:_____

Wins:_____

Challenges:_____

Comments:_____

_____

_____

_____

_____

_____

One Word   Success Score (1-10)

DAY 15
WEEK 3

DATE ___/___/___

Energy:	"Big M":	Health:	Mood:	Stress:

DIET   Success Score:_____

Meals:_____

_____

_____

_____

_____

DATA

Weight:	Fat %:	x1: _____	x2: _____

MACRONUTRIENT CALCULATIONS

Carbs:	Protein:	Fat:	Calories:

_____

_____

_____

_____

Snacks:_____

_____

Comments:_____

_____

_____

_____

PRIMAL LIFESTYLE   Success Score:_____

Sleep (1-10):_____   Comments:_____

Sun (1-10):_____   Comments:_____

Play (1-10):_____   Comments:_____

Brain (1-10):_____   Comments:_____

Move (1-10):_____   Comments:_____

PERSONAL

Comments:_____

_____

_____

_____

EXERCISE   Success Score:_____   Effort Score:_____

Workout:_____

Location:_____ Duration:_____

Exercise 1:_____ Weight:_____ Reps/Time:_____ Set 2:_____ Set 3:_____

Exercise 2:_____ Weight:_____ Reps/Time:_____ Set 2:_____ Set 3:_____

Exercise 3:_____ Weight:_____ Reps/Time:_____ Set 2:_____ Set 3:_____

Exercise 4:_____ Weight:_____ Reps/Time:_____ Set 2:_____ Set 3:_____

Exercise 5:_____ Weight:_____ Reps/Time:_____ Set 2:_____ Set 3:_____

Exercise 6:_____ Weight:_____ Reps/Time:_____ Set 2:_____ Set 3:_____

Comments:_____

_____

_____

_____

_____

Workout:_____

Location:_____ Distance:_____ Duration:_____

Comments:_____

_____

_____

_____

SUMMARY

Tomorrow:_____

This Week:_____ This Month:_____

Wins:_____

Challenges:_____

Comments:_____

_____

_____

_____

_____

One Word   Success Score (1-10)

DAY 16
WEEK 3

DATE
/ /

Energy:	"Big M":	Health:	Mood:	Stress:

DIET
Success Score:_____

Meals:_____

_____

_____

_____

_____

DATA

Weight:	Fat %:	x1: _____	x2: _____

MACRONUTRIENT CALCULATIONS

Carbs:	Protein:	Fat:	Calories:

_____

_____

_____

_____

Snacks:_____

_____

Comments:_____

_____

_____

_____

PRIMAL LIFESTYLE
Success Score:_____

Sleep (1-10):_____ Comments:_____

Sun (1-10):_____ Comments:_____

Play (1-10):_____ Comments:_____

Brain (1-10):_____ Comments:_____

Move (1-10):_____ Comments:_____

PERSONAL

Comments:_____

_____

_____

_____

EXERCISE   Success Score:_____   Effort Score:_____

Workout:_____

Location:_____ Duration:_____

Exercise 1:_____ Weight:_____ Reps/Time:_____ Set 2:_____ Set 3:_____

Exercise 2:_____ Weight:_____ Reps/Time:_____ Set 2:_____ Set 3:_____

Exercise 3:_____ Weight:_____ Reps/Time:_____ Set 2:_____ Set 3:_____

Exercise 4:_____ Weight:_____ Reps/Time:_____ Set 2:_____ Set 3:_____

Exercise 5:_____ Weight:_____ Reps/Time:_____ Set 2:_____ Set 3:_____

Exercise 6:_____ Weight:_____ Reps/Time:_____ Set 2:_____ Set 3:_____

Comments:_____

_____

_____

_____

_____

Workout:_____

Location:_____ Distance:_____ Duration:_____

Comments:_____

_____

_____

_____

_____

SUMMARY

Tomorrow:_____

This Week:_____ This Month:_____

Wins:_____

Challenges:_____

Comments:_____

_____

_____

_____

_____

One Word   Success Score (1-10)

DAY 17
WEEK 3

1 - 10 SCORE

Energy:	"Big M":	Health:	Mood:	Stress:

DIET

Success Score:_____

Meals:_____

_____

_____

_____

DATA

Weight:	Fat %:	x1: _____	x2: _____

MACRONUTRIENT CALCULATIONS

Carbs:	Protein:	Fat:	Calories:

_____

_____

_____

_____

Snacks:_____

_____

Comments:_____

_____

_____

_____

PRIMAL LIFESTYLE

Success Score:_____

Sleep (1-10):_____   Comments:_____

Sun (1-10):_____   Comments:_____

Play (1-10):_____   Comments:_____

Brain (1-10):_____   Comments:_____

Move (1-10):_____   Comments:_____

PERSONAL

Comments:_____

_____

_____

_____

EXERCISE Success Score:_____ Effort Score:_____

Workout:_____

Location:_____ Duration:_____

Exercise 1:_____ Weight:_____ Reps/Time:_____ Set 2:_____ Set 3:_____

Exercise 2:_____ Weight:_____ Reps/Time:_____ Set 2:_____ Set 3:_____

Exercise 3:_____ Weight:_____ Reps/Time:_____ Set 2:_____ Set 3:_____

Exercise 4:_____ Weight:_____ Reps/Time:_____ Set 2:_____ Set 3:_____

Exercise 5:_____ Weight:_____ Reps/Time:_____ Set 2:_____ Set 3:_____

Exercise 6:_____ Weight:_____ Reps/Time:_____ Set 2:_____ Set 3:_____

Comments:_____

_____

_____

_____

_____

Workout:_____

Location:_____ Distance:_____ Duration:_____

Comments:_____

_____

_____

_____

_____

SUMMARY

Tomorrow:_____

This Week:_____ This Month:_____

Wins:_____

Challenges:_____

Comments:_____

_____

_____

_____

_____

_____

One Word   Success Score (1-10)

DAY 18
WEEK 3

DATE / /

1 - 10 SCORE

Energy:	"Big M":	Health:	Mood:	Stress:

DIET   Success Score:_____

Meals:_____

_____

DATA

Weight:	Fat %:	x1: _____	x2: _____

MACRONUTRIENT CALCULATIONS

Carbs:	Protein:	Fat:	Calories:

_____

_____

_____

_____

Snacks:_____

_____

Comments:_____

_____

_____

_____

PRIMAL LIFESTYLE   Success Score:_____

Sleep (1-10):_____   Comments:_____

Sun (1-10):_____   Comments:_____

Play (1-10):_____   Comments:_____

Brain (1-10):_____   Comments:_____

Move (1-10):_____   Comments:_____

PERSONAL

Comments:_____

_____

_____

_____

EXERCISE   Success Score:_____   Effort Score:_____

Workout:_____

Location:_____ Duration:_____

Exercise 1:_____ Weight:_____ Reps/Time:_____ Set 2:_____ Set 3:_____

Exercise 2:_____ Weight:_____ Reps/Time:_____ Set 2:_____ Set 3:_____

Exercise 3:_____ Weight:_____ Reps/Time:_____ Set 2:_____ Set 3:_____

Exercise 4:_____ Weight:_____ Reps/Time:_____ Set 2:_____ Set 3:_____

Exercise 5:_____ Weight:_____ Reps/Time:_____ Set 2:_____ Set 3:_____

Exercise 6:_____ Weight:_____ Reps/Time:_____ Set 2:_____ Set 3:_____

Comments:_____

_____

_____

_____

_____

Workout:_____

Location:_____ Distance:_____ Duration:_____

Comments:_____

_____

_____

_____

SUMMARY

Tomorrow:_____

This Week:_____ This Month:_____

Wins:_____

Challenges:_____

Comments:_____

_____

_____

_____

_____

_____

One Word   Success Score (1-10)

DAY 19
WEEK 3

DATE
/ /

1 - 10 SCORE

Energy:	"Big M":	Health:	Mood:	Stress:

DIET

Success Score:_____

Meals:_____

_____

_____

_____

_____

DATA

Weight:	Fat %:	x1: _____	x2: _____

MACRONUTRIENT CALCULATIONS

Carbs:	Protein:	Fat:	Calories:

_____

_____

_____

_____

Snacks:_____

_____

Comments:_____

_____

_____

_____

PRIMAL LIFESTYLE

Success Score:_____

Sleep (1-10):_____   Comments:_____

Sun (1-10):_____   Comments:_____

Play (1-10):_____   Comments:_____

Brain (1-10):_____   Comments:_____

Move (1-10):_____   Comments:_____

PERSONAL

Comments:_____

_____

_____

_____

EXERCISE   Success Score:_____   Effort Score:_____

Workout:_____

Location:_____   Duration:_____

Exercise 1:_____ Weight:_____ Reps/Time:_____ Set 2:_____ Set 3:_____

Exercise 2:_____ Weight:_____ Reps/Time:_____ Set 2:_____ Set 3:_____

Exercise 3:_____ Weight:_____ Reps/Time:_____ Set 2:_____ Set 3:_____

Exercise 4:_____ Weight:_____ Reps/Time:_____ Set 2:_____ Set 3:_____

Exercise 5:_____ Weight:_____ Reps/Time:_____ Set 2:_____ Set 3:_____

Exercise 6:_____ Weight:_____ Reps/Time:_____ Set 2:_____ Set 3:_____

Comments:_____

_____

_____

_____

Workout:_____

Location:_____ Distance:_____ Duration:_____

Comments:_____

_____

_____

_____

SUMMARY

Tomorrow:_____

This Week:_____ This Month:_____

Wins:_____

Challenges:_____

Comments:_____

_____

_____

_____

_____

_____

One Word   Success Score (1-10)

DAY 20
WEEK 3

DATE ___ / ___ / ___

1 - 10 SCORE

Energy:	"Big M":	Health:	Mood:	Stress:

DIET

Success Score:_____

Meals:_____

_____

_____

_____

DATA

Weight:	Fat %:	x1: _____	x2: _____

MACRONUTRIENT CALCULATIONS

Carbs:	Protein:	Fat:	Calories:

_____

_____

_____

_____

Snacks:_____

Comments:_____

_____

_____

_____

PRIMAL LIFESTYLE

Success Score:_____

Sleep (1-10):_____ Comments:_____

Sun (1-10):_____ Comments:_____

Play (1-10):_____ Comments:_____

Brain (1-10):_____ Comments:_____

Move (1-10):_____ Comments:_____

PERSONAL

Comments:_____

_____

_____

_____

EXERCISE   Success Score:_____   Effort Score:_____

Workout:_____

Location:_____ Duration:_____

Exercise 1:_____Weight:_____Reps/Time:_____Set 2:_____Set 3:_____

Exercise 2:_____Weight:_____Reps/Time:_____Set 2:_____Set 3:_____

Exercise 3:_____Weight:_____Reps/Time:_____Set 2:_____Set 3:_____

Exercise 4:_____Weight:_____Reps/Time:_____Set 2:_____Set 3:_____

Exercise 5:_____Weight:_____Reps/Time:_____Set 2:_____Set 3:_____

Exercise 6:_____Weight:_____Reps/Time:_____Set 2:_____Set 3:_____

Comments:_____

_____

_____

_____

_____

Workout:_____

Location:_____ Distance:_____ Duration:_____

Comments:_____

_____

_____

_____

SUMMARY

Tomorrow:_____

This Week:_____ This Month:_____

Wins:_____

Challenges:_____

Comments:_____

_____

_____

_____

_____

_____

One Word   Success Score (1-10)

DAY 21
WEEK 3

1 - 10 SCORE

Energy:	"Big M":	Health:	Mood:	Stress:

DIET

Success Score:_____

Meals:_____

_____

_____

_____

DATA

Weight:	Fat %:	x1: _____	x2: _____

MACRONUTRIENT CALCULATIONS

Carbs:	Protein:	Fat:	Calories:

_____

_____

_____

_____

Snacks:_____

Comments:_____

_____

_____

_____

PRIMAL LIFESTYLE

Success Score:_____

Sleep (1-10):_____ Comments:_____

Sun (1-10):_____ Comments:_____

Play (1-10):_____ Comments:_____

Brain (1-10):_____ Comments:_____

Move (1-10):_____ Comments:_____

PERSONAL

Comments:_____

_____

_____

_____

EXERCISE   Success Score:_____   Effort Score:_____

Workout:_____

Location:_____ Duration:_____

Exercise 1:_____ Weight:_____ Reps/Time:_____ Set 2:_____ Set 3:_____

Exercise 2:_____ Weight:_____ Reps/Time:_____ Set 2:_____ Set 3:_____

Exercise 3:_____ Weight:_____ Reps/Time:_____ Set 2:_____ Set 3:_____

Exercise 4:_____ Weight:_____ Reps/Time:_____ Set 2:_____ Set 3:_____

Exercise 5:_____ Weight:_____ Reps/Time:_____ Set 2:_____ Set 3:_____

Exercise 6:_____ Weight:_____ Reps/Time:_____ Set 2:_____ Set 3:_____

Comments:_____

_____

_____

_____

_____

Workout:_____

Location:_____ Distance:_____ Duration:_____

Comments:_____

_____

_____

_____

_____

SUMMARY

Tomorrow:_____

This Week:_____ This Month:_____

Wins:_____

Challenges:_____

Comments:_____

_____

_____

_____

_____

_____

One Word   Success Score (1-10)

DAY 22
WEEK 4

DATE
/ /

1 - 10 SCORE

Energy:	"Big M":	Health:	Mood:	Stress:

DIET

Success Score:_____

Meals:_____

_____

_____

_____

_____

DATA

Weight:	Fat %:	x1: _____	x2: _____

MACRONUTRIENT CALCULATIONS

Carbs:	Protein:	Fat:	Calories:

_____

_____

_____

_____

Snacks:_____

_____

Comments:_____

_____

_____

_____

PRIMAL LIFESTYLE

Success Score:_____

Sleep (1-10):_____ Comments:_____

Sun (1-10):_____ Comments:_____

Play (1-10):_____ Comments:_____

Brain (1-10):_____ Comments:_____

Move (1-10):_____ Comments:_____

PERSONAL

Comments:_____

_____

_____

_____

EXERCISE   Success Score:_____   Effort Score:_____

Workout:_____

Location:_____ Duration:_____

Exercise 1:_____Weight:_____ Reps/Time:_____Set 2:_____Set 3:_____

Exercise 2:_____Weight:_____ Reps/Time:_____Set 2:_____Set 3:_____

Exercise 3:_____Weight:_____ Reps/Time:_____Set 2:_____Set 3:_____

Exercise 4:_____Weight:_____ Reps/Time:_____Set 2:_____Set 3:_____

Exercise 5:_____Weight:_____ Reps/Time:_____Set 2:_____Set 3:_____

Exercise 6:_____Weight:_____ Reps/Time:_____Set 2:_____Set 3:_____

Comments:_____

_____

_____

_____

_____

Workout:_____

Location:_____ Distance:_____ Duration:_____

Comments:_____

_____

_____

_____

_____

SUMMARY

Tomorrow:_____

This Week:_____ This Month:_____

Wins:_____

Challenges:_____

Comments:_____

_____

_____

_____

_____

_____

One Word   Success Score (1-10)

DAY 23
WEEK 4

DATE / /

1 - 10 SCORE

Energy:	"Big M":	Health:	Mood:	Stress:

DIET

Success Score:_____

DATA

Weight:	Fat %:	x1: _____	x2: _____

Meals:_____

_____

MACRONUTRIENT CALCULATIONS

Carbs:	Protein:	Fat:	Calories:

_____

_____

_____

_____

_____

_____

_____

Snacks:_____

_____

Comments:_____

_____

_____

_____

PRIMAL LIFESTYLE

Success Score:_____

Sleep (1-10):_____ Comments:_____

Sun (1-10):_____ Comments:_____

Play (1-10):_____ Comments:_____

Brain (1-10):_____ Comments:_____

Move (1-10):_____ Comments:_____

PERSONAL

Comments:_____

_____

_____

_____

EXERCISE   Success Score:_____   Effort Score:_____

Workout:_____

Location:_____ Duration:_____

Exercise 1:_____Weight:_____ Reps/Time:_____ Set 2:_____ Set 3:_____

Exercise 2:_____Weight:_____ Reps/Time:_____ Set 2:_____ Set 3:_____

Exercise 3:_____Weight:_____ Reps/Time:_____ Set 2:_____ Set 3:_____

Exercise 4:_____Weight:_____ Reps/Time:_____ Set 2:_____ Set 3:_____

Exercise 5:_____Weight:_____ Reps/Time:_____ Set 2:_____ Set 3:_____

Exercise 6:_____Weight:_____ Reps/Time:_____ Set 2:_____ Set 3:_____

Comments:_____

_____

_____

_____

_____

Workout:_____

Location:_____ Distance:_____ Duration:_____

Comments:_____

_____

_____

_____

SUMMARY

Tomorrow:_____

This Week:_____ This Month:_____

Wins:_____

Challenges:_____

Comments:_____

_____

_____

_____

_____

_____

One Word   Success Score (1-10)

DAY 24
WEEK 4

DATE __ / __ / __

1 - 10 SCORE

Energy:	"Big M":	Health:	Mood:	Stress:

DIET

Success Score:_____

Meals:_____

_____

_____

_____

DATA

Weight:	Fat %:	x1: _____	x2: _____

MACRONUTRIENT CALCULATIONS

Carbs:	Protein:	Fat:	Calories:

_____

_____

_____

_____

Snacks:_____

_____

Comments:_____

_____

_____

_____

PRIMAL LIFESTYLE

Success Score:_____

Sleep (1-10):_____ Comments:_____

Sun (1-10):_____ Comments:_____

Play (1-10):_____ Comments:_____

Brain (1-10):_____ Comments:_____

Move (1-10):_____ Comments:_____

PERSONAL

Comments:_____

_____

_____

_____

EXERCISE   Success Score:_____   Effort Score:_____

Workout:_____

Location:_____   Duration:_____

Exercise 1:_____ Weight:_____ Reps/Time:_____ Set 2:_____ Set 3:_____

Exercise 2:_____ Weight:_____ Reps/Time:_____ Set 2:_____ Set 3:_____

Exercise 3:_____ Weight:_____ Reps/Time:_____ Set 2:_____ Set 3:_____

Exercise 4:_____ Weight:_____ Reps/Time:_____ Set 2:_____ Set 3:_____

Exercise 5:_____ Weight:_____ Reps/Time:_____ Set 2:_____ Set 3:_____

Exercise 6:_____ Weight:_____ Reps/Time:_____ Set 2:_____ Set 3:_____

Comments:_____

_____

_____

_____

_____

Workout:_____

Location:_____ Distance:_____ Duration:_____

Comments:_____

_____

_____

_____

_____

SUMMARY

Tomorrow:_____

This Week:_____   This Month:_____

Wins:_____

Challenges:_____

Comments:_____

_____

_____

_____

_____

_____

One Word   Success Score (1-10)

DAY 25
WEEK 4

DATE
/ /

1 - 10 SCORE

Energy:	"Big M":	Health:	Mood:	Stress:

DIET

Success Score:_____

Meals:_____
_____
_____
_____

DATA

Weight:	Fat %:	x1: _____	x2: _____

MACRONUTRIENT CALCULATIONS

Carbs:	Protein:	Fat:	Calories:

_____
_____
_____
_____

Snacks:_____
_____

Comments:_____
_____
_____
_____

PRIMAL LIFESTYLE

Success Score:_____

Sleep (1-10):_____   Comments:_____
Sun (1-10):_____   Comments:_____
Play (1-10):_____   Comments:_____
Brain (1-10):_____   Comments:_____
Move (1-10):_____   Comments:_____

PERSONAL

Comments:_____
_____
_____
_____

EXERCISE   Success Score:_____   Effort Score:_____

Workout:_____

Location:_____   Duration:_____

Exercise 1:_____Weight:_____Reps/Time:_____Set 2:_____Set 3:_____

Exercise 2:_____Weight:_____Reps/Time:_____Set 2:_____Set 3:_____

Exercise 3:_____Weight:_____Reps/Time:_____Set 2:_____Set 3:_____

Exercise 4:_____Weight:_____Reps/Time:_____Set 2:_____Set 3:_____

Exercise 5:_____Weight:_____Reps/Time:_____Set 2:_____Set 3:_____

Exercise 6:_____Weight:_____Reps/Time:_____Set 2:_____Set 3:_____

Comments:_____

_____

_____

_____

_____

Workout:_____

Location:_____   Distance:_____   Duration:_____

Comments:_____

_____

_____

_____

_____

SUMMARY

Tomorrow:_____

This Week:_____   This Month:_____

Wins:_____

Challenges:_____

Comments:_____

_____

_____

_____

_____

_____

One Word	Success Score (1-10)

DAY 26
WEEK 4

DATE ___/___/___

1 - 10 SCORE

Energy:	"Big M":	Health:	Mood:	Stress:

DIET   Success Score:_____

Meals:_____

_____

_____

_____

DATA

Weight:	Fat %:	$x1$: _____	$x2$: _____

MACRONUTRIENT CALCULATIONS

Carbs:	Protein:	Fat:	Calories:

_____

_____

_____

_____

Snacks:_____

_____

Comments:_____

_____

_____

_____

PRIMAL LIFESTYLE   Success Score:_____

Sleep (1-10):_____ Comments:_____

Sun (1-10):_____ Comments:_____

Play (1-10):_____ Comments:_____

Brain (1-10):_____ Comments:_____

Move (1-10):_____ Comments:_____

PERSONAL

Comments:_____

_____

_____

_____

EXERCISE   Success Score:_____   Effort Score:_____

Workout:_____

Location:_____ Duration:_____

Exercise 1:_____Weight:_____Reps/Time:_____Set 2:_____Set 3:_____

Exercise 2:_____Weight:_____Reps/Time:_____Set 2:_____Set 3:_____

Exercise 3:_____Weight:_____Reps/Time:_____Set 2:_____Set 3:_____

Exercise 4:_____Weight:_____Reps/Time:_____Set 2:_____Set 3:_____

Exercise 5:_____Weight:_____Reps/Time:_____Set 2:_____Set 3:_____

Exercise 6:_____Weight:_____Reps/Time:_____Set 2:_____Set 3:_____

Comments:_____

_____

_____

_____

_____

Workout:_____

Location:_____ Distance:_____ Duration:_____

Comments:_____

_____

_____

_____

_____

SUMMARY

Tomorrow:_____

This Week:_____ This Month:_____

Wins:_____

Challenges:_____

Comments:_____

_____

_____

_____

_____

One Word   Success Score (1-10)

DAY 27
WEEK 4

DATE
/ /

1 - 10 SCORE

Energy:	"Big M":	Health:	Mood:	Stress:

DIET

Success Score:_____

Meals:_____

_____

_____

_____

_____

DATA

Weight:	Fat %:	x1: _____	x2: _____

MACRONUTRIENT CALCULATIONS

Carbs:	Protein:	Fat:	Calories:

_____

_____

_____

_____

Snacks:_____

_____

Comments:_____

_____

_____

_____

PRIMAL LIFESTYLE

Success Score:_____

Sleep (1-10):_____   Comments:_____

Sun (1-10):_____   Comments:_____

Play (1-10):_____   Comments:_____

Brain (1-10):_____   Comments:_____

Move (1-10):_____   Comments:_____

PERSONAL

Comments:_____

_____

_____

_____

EXERCISE   Success Score:_____   Effort Score:_____

Workout:_____

Location:_____ Duration:_____

Exercise 1:_____Weight:_____Reps/Time:_____Set 2:_____Set 3:_____

Exercise 2:_____Weight:_____Reps/Time:_____Set 2:_____Set 3:_____

Exercise 3:_____Weight:_____Reps/Time:_____Set 2:_____Set 3:_____

Exercise 4:_____Weight:_____Reps/Time:_____Set 2:_____Set 3:_____

Exercise 5:_____Weight:_____Reps/Time:_____Set 2:_____Set 3:_____

Exercise 6:_____Weight:_____Reps/Time:_____Set 2:_____Set 3:_____

Comments:_____

_____

_____

_____

_____

Workout:_____

Location:_____ Distance:_____ Duration:_____

Comments:_____

_____

_____

_____

_____

SUMMARY

Tomorrow:_____

This Week:_____ This Month:_____

Wins:_____

Challenges:_____

Comments:_____

_____

_____

_____

_____

_____

| One Word | Success Score (1-10) |

DAY 28
WEEK 4

DATE ___/___/___

1 - 10 SCORE

Energy:	"Big M":	Health:	Mood:	Stress:

DIET   Success Score:_____

Meals:_____

_____

_____

_____

_____

DATA

Weight:	Fat %:	x1: _____	x2: _____

MACRONUTRIENT CALCULATIONS

Carbs:	Protein:	Fat:	Calories:

_____

_____

_____

_____

Snacks:_____

_____

Comments:_____

_____

_____

_____

PRIMAL LIFESTYLE   Success Score:_____

Sleep (1-10):_____   Comments:_____

Sun (1-10):_____   Comments:_____

Play (1-10):_____   Comments:_____

Brain (1-10):_____   Comments:_____

Move (1-10):_____   Comments:_____

PERSONAL

Comments:_____

_____

_____

_____

EXERCISE   Success Score:_____   Effort Score:_____

Workout:_____

Location:_____   Duration:_____

Exercise 1:_____ Weight:_____ Reps/Time:_____ Set 2:_____ Set 3:_____
Exercise 2:_____ Weight:_____ Reps/Time:_____ Set 2:_____ Set 3:_____
Exercise 3:_____ Weight:_____ Reps/Time:_____ Set 2:_____ Set 3:_____
Exercise 4:_____ Weight:_____ Reps/Time:_____ Set 2:_____ Set 3:_____
Exercise 5:_____ Weight:_____ Reps/Time:_____ Set 2:_____ Set 3:_____
Exercise 6:_____ Weight:_____ Reps/Time:_____ Set 2:_____ Set 3:_____

Comments:_____

_____

_____

_____

_____

Workout:_____

Location:_____ Distance:_____ Duration:_____

Comments:_____

_____

_____

_____

SUMMARY

Tomorrow:_____

This Week:_____ This Month:_____

Wins:_____

Challenges:_____

Comments:_____

_____

_____

_____

_____

One Word   Success Score (1-10)

DAY 29
WEEK 5

DATE / /

1 - 10 SCORE

Energy:	"Big M":	Health:	Mood:	Stress:

DIET   Success Score:_____

Meals:_____
_____
_____
_____
_____

DATA

Weight:	Fat %:	x1: _____	x2: _____

MACRONUTRIENT CALCULATIONS

Carbs:	Protein:	Fat:	Calories:

_____
_____
_____
_____

Snacks:_____
_____

Comments:_____
_____
_____
_____

PRIMAL LIFESTYLE   Success Score:_____

Sleep (1-10):_____   Comments:_____
Sun (1-10):_____   Comments:_____
Play (1-10):_____   Comments:_____
Brain (1-10):_____   Comments:_____
Move (1-10):_____   Comments:_____

PERSONAL

Comments:_____
_____
_____
_____

EXERCISE   Success Score:_____   Effort Score:_____

Workout:_____

Location:_____ Duration:_____

Exercise 1:_____Weight:_____Reps/Time:_____Set 2:_____Set 3:_____

Exercise 2:_____Weight:_____Reps/Time:_____Set 2:_____Set 3:_____

Exercise 3:_____Weight:_____Reps/Time:_____Set 2:_____Set 3:_____

Exercise 4:_____Weight:_____Reps/Time:_____Set 2:_____Set 3:_____

Exercise 5:_____Weight:_____Reps/Time:_____Set 2:_____Set 3:_____

Exercise 6:_____Weight:_____Reps/Time:_____Set 2:_____Set 3:_____

Comments:_____

_____

_____

_____

_____

Workout:_____

Location:_____ Distance:_____ Duration:_____

Comments:_____

_____

_____

_____

SUMMARY

Tomorrow:_____

This Week:_____ This Month:_____

Wins:_____

Challenges:_____

Comments:_____

_____

_____

_____

One Word   Success Score (1-10)

DAY 30
WEEK 5

DATE
/ /

1 - 10 SCORE

Energy:	"Big M":	Health:	Mood:	Stress:

DIET

Success Score:_____

Meals:_____

_____

_____

_____

DATA

Weight:	Fat %:	x1: _____	x2: _____

MACRONUTRIENT CALCULATIONS

Carbs:	Protein:	Fat:	Calories:

_____

_____

_____

_____

Snacks:_____

_____

Comments:_____

_____

_____

_____

PRIMAL LIFESTYLE

Success Score:_____

Sleep (1-10):_____ Comments:_____

Sun (1-10):_____ Comments:_____

Play (1-10):_____ Comments:_____

Brain (1-10):_____ Comments:_____

Move (1-10):_____ Comments:_____

PERSONAL

Comments:_____

_____

_____

_____

EXERCISE   Success Score:_____   Effort Score:_____

Workout:_____

Location:_____ Duration:_____

Exercise 1:_____Weight:_____Reps/Time:_____Set 2:_____Set 3:_____

Exercise 2:_____Weight:_____Reps/Time:_____Set 2:_____Set 3:_____

Exercise 3:_____Weight:_____Reps/Time:_____Set 2:_____Set 3:_____

Exercise 4:_____Weight:_____Reps/Time:_____Set 2:_____Set 3:_____

Exercise 5:_____Weight:_____Reps/Time:_____Set 2:_____Set 3:_____

Exercise 6:_____Weight:_____Reps/Time:_____Set 2:_____Set 3:_____

Comments:_____

_____

_____

_____

_____

Workout:_____

Location:_____ Distance:_____ Duration:_____

Comments:_____

_____

_____

_____

SUMMARY

Tomorrow:_____

This Week:_____ This Month:_____

Wins:_____

Challenges:_____

Comments:_____

_____

_____

_____

_____

One Word   Success Score (1-10)

DAY 30 EVALUATION

/ / DATE

DIET
Past 30 days.

Success Score:_____

Wins:_____

Challenges:_____

Comments:_____

_____

_____

_____

_____

1 - 10 SCORE

Energy:	"Big M":	Health:	Mood:	Stress:

MACRONUTRIENT CALCULATIONS

Carbs:	Protein:	Fat:	Calories:

PRIMAL LIFESTYLE
Past 30 days.

Success Score:_____

Sleep (1-10):_____ Comments:_____

Sun (1-10):_____ Comments:_____

Play (1-10):_____ Comments:_____

Brain (1-10):_____ Comments:_____

Move (1-10):_____ Comments:_____

PERSONAL
Past 30 days.

Comments:_____

_____

_____

_____

_____

_____

_____

DAY 30 EVALUATION

Past 30 days.

Success Score:_____ Effort Score:_____

Wins:_____

Challenges:_____

Comments:_____

_____

_____

_____

GOALS

1._____

2._____

3._____

4._____

5._____

BODY MEASUREMENTS

Time of Day:_____ Scale/method used:_____

Day 1 weight:_____ Day 1 fat %:_____

Day 2 weight:_____ Day 2 fat %:_____

Day 3 weight:_____ Day 3 fat %:_____

Average weight:_____ Average body fat %:_____

Body part measurements:.

Waistline:_____ Hips:_____ Chest:_____

Thighs:_____ Biceps:_____

Other body measurement:_____ Value:_____

Other body measurement:_____ Value:_____

DAY 30 EVALUATION

FITNESS MEASUREMENTS

Morning resting heart rate:_____ _____ _____ Average:_____
                             Day 1   Day 2   Day 3

Primal Essential Movements – one set maximum effort

Note type of progression or advanced exercise if not actual Essential Movement
(e.g. – decline pushups, chair-assisted pullups)

Pushups:_____ Number:_____

Pullups:_____ Number:_____

Squats:_____ Number:_____

Plank:_____ Time:_____

400-meter run:_____ Date:_____

Location/conditions/notes:_____

One-mile run:_____ Date:_____

Location/conditions/notes:_____

_____

Maximum Aerobic Function test

Date:_____ Heart Rate:_____

Course/distance:_____ Time:_____

Location/conditions/notes:_____

VO2 Max test (ml/kg value):_____

Date/location/method of test:_____

Other best performances:

Event/Exercise:_____Achievement:_____

Event/Exercise:_____Achievement:_____

Event/Exercise:_____Achievement:_____

"I don't claim to be perfect;
but I'm a hell of a lot better off
than I've ever been before.
I live by my own 85/15 rule that
seems to feel right for my body;
The Primal lifestyle is not always
about losing. It can be about
gaining too; gaining health, happiness,
and yes, even weight when you need to."

– Success Story Katie

DAY 31
WEEK 5

DATE ___ / ___ / ___

1 - 10 SCORE

Energy:	"Big M":	Health:	Mood:	Stress:

DIET   Success Score:_____

Meals:_____

_____

_____

_____

DATA

Weight:	Fat %:	x1: _____	x2: _____

MACRONUTRIENT CALCULATIONS

Carbs:	Protein:	Fat:	Calories:

_____

_____

_____

_____

Snacks:_____

_____

Comments:_____

_____

_____

_____

PRIMAL LIFESTYLE   Success Score:_____

Sleep (1-10):_____   Comments:_____

Sun (1-10):_____   Comments:_____

Play (1-10):_____   Comments:_____

Brain (1-10):_____   Comments:_____

Move (1-10):_____   Comments:_____

PERSONAL

Comments:_____

_____

_____

_____

EXERCISE   Success Score:_____   Effort Score:_____

Workout:_____

Location:_____   Duration:_____

Exercise 1:_____Weight:_____Reps/Time:_____Set 2:_____Set 3:_____

Exercise 2:_____Weight:_____Reps/Time:_____Set 2:_____Set 3:_____

Exercise 3:_____Weight:_____Reps/Time:_____Set 2:_____Set 3:_____

Exercise 4:_____Weight:_____Reps/Time:_____Set 2:_____Set 3:_____

Exercise 5:_____Weight:_____Reps/Time:_____Set 2:_____Set 3:_____

Exercise 6:_____Weight:_____Reps/Time:_____Set 2:_____Set 3:_____

Comments:_____
_____
_____
_____
_____

Workout:_____

Location:_____   Distance:_____   Duration:_____

Comments:_____
_____
_____
_____
_____

SUMMARY

Tomorrow:_____

This Week:_____   This Month:_____

Wins:_____

Challenges:_____

Comments:_____
_____
_____
_____
_____
_____

One Word   Success Score (1-10)

DAY 32
WEEK 5

DATE
/ /

Energy:	"Big M":	Health:	Mood:	Stress:

DIET

Success Score:_____

Meals:_____

_____

_____

_____

DATA

Weight:	Fat %:	x1: _____	x2: _____

MACRONUTRIENT CALCULATIONS

Carbs:	Protein:	Fat:	Calories:

_____

_____

_____

_____

Snacks:_____

_____

Comments:_____

_____

_____

_____

PRIMAL LIFESTYLE

Success Score:_____

Sleep (1-10):_____ Comments:_____

Sun (1-10):_____ Comments:_____

Play (1-10):_____ Comments:_____

Brain (1-10):_____ Comments:_____

Move (1-10):_____ Comments:_____

PERSONAL

Comments:_____

_____

_____

_____

EXERCISE   Success Score:_____   Effort Score:_____

Workout:_____

Location:_____ Duration:_____

Exercise 1:_____	Weight:_____	Reps/Time:_____	Set 2:_____	Set 3:_____
Exercise 2:_____	Weight:_____	Reps/Time:_____	Set 2:_____	Set 3:_____
Exercise 3:_____	Weight:_____	Reps/Time:_____	Set 2:_____	Set 3:_____
Exercise 4:_____	Weight:_____	Reps/Time:_____	Set 2:_____	Set 3:_____
Exercise 5:_____	Weight:_____	Reps/Time:_____	Set 2:_____	Set 3:_____
Exercise 6:_____	Weight:_____	Reps/Time:_____	Set 2:_____	Set 3:_____

Comments:_____
_____
_____
_____
_____

Workout:_____

Location:_____ Distance:_____ Duration:_____

Comments:_____
_____
_____
_____

SUMMARY

Tomorrow:_____

This Week:_____ This Month:_____

Wins:_____

Challenges:_____

Comments:_____
_____
_____
_____
_____

One Word   Success Score (1-10)

DAY 33
WEEK 5

DATE / /

1 - 10 SCORE

Energy:	"Big M":	Health:	Mood:	Stress:

DIET   Success Score:_____

Meals:_____

_____

_____

_____

_____

DATA

Weight:	Fat %:	x1: _____	x2: _____

MACRONUTRIENT CALCULATIONS

Carbs:	Protein:	Fat:	Calories:

_____

_____

_____

_____

Snacks:_____

_____

Comments:_____

_____

_____

_____

PRIMAL LIFESTYLE   Success Score:_____

Sleep (1-10):_____ Comments:_____

Sun (1-10):_____ Comments:_____

Play (1-10):_____ Comments:_____

Brain (1-10):_____ Comments:_____

Move (1-10):_____ Comments:_____

PERSONAL

Comments:_____

_____

_____

_____

EXERCISE   Success Score:_____   Effort Score:_____

Workout:_____

Location:_____   Duration:_____

Exercise 1:_____	Weight:_____	Reps/Time:_____	Set 2:_____	Set 3:_____
Exercise 2:_____	Weight:_____	Reps/Time:_____	Set 2:_____	Set 3:_____
Exercise 3:_____	Weight:_____	Reps/Time:_____	Set 2:_____	Set 3:_____
Exercise 4:_____	Weight:_____	Reps/Time:_____	Set 2:_____	Set 3:_____
Exercise 5:_____	Weight:_____	Reps/Time:_____	Set 2:_____	Set 3:_____
Exercise 6:_____	Weight:_____	Reps/Time:_____	Set 2:_____	Set 3:_____

Comments:_____

_____

_____

_____

_____

Workout:_____

Location:_____   Distance:_____   Duration:_____

Comments:_____

_____

_____

_____

_____

SUMMARY

Tomorrow:_____

This Week:_____   This Month:_____

Wins:_____

Challenges:_____

Comments:_____

_____

_____

_____

_____   [   ]   [   ]

_____   One Word   Success Score (1-10)

DAY 34
WEEK 5

DATE

/ /

1 - 10 SCORE

Energy:	"Big M":	Health:	Mood:	Stress:

DIET

Success Score:_____

Meals:_____

_____

_____

_____

DATA

Weight:	Fat %:	x1: _____	x2: _____

MACRONUTRIENT CALCULATIONS

Carbs:	Protein:	Fat:	Calories:

_____

_____

_____

_____

Snacks:_____

_____

Comments:_____

_____

_____

_____

PRIMAL LIFESTYLE

Success Score:_____

Sleep (1-10):_____ Comments:_____

Sun (1-10):_____ Comments:_____

Play (1-10):_____ Comments:_____

Brain (1-10):_____ Comments:_____

Move (1-10):_____ Comments:_____

PERSONAL

Comments:_____

_____

_____

_____

EXERCISE   Success Score:_____   Effort Score:_____

Workout:_____

Location:_____ Duration:_____

Exercise 1:_____ Weight:_____ Reps/Time:_____ Set 2:_____ Set 3:_____

Exercise 2:_____ Weight:_____ Reps/Time:_____ Set 2:_____ Set 3:_____

Exercise 3:_____ Weight:_____ Reps/Time:_____ Set 2:_____ Set 3:_____

Exercise 4:_____ Weight:_____ Reps/Time:_____ Set 2:_____ Set 3:_____

Exercise 5:_____ Weight:_____ Reps/Time:_____ Set 2:_____ Set 3:_____

Exercise 6:_____ Weight:_____ Reps/Time:_____ Set 2:_____ Set 3:_____

Comments:_____

_____

_____

_____

_____

Workout:_____

Location:_____ Distance:_____ Duration:_____

Comments:_____

_____

_____

_____

_____

SUMMARY

Tomorrow:_____

This Week:_____ This Month:_____

Wins:_____

Challenges:_____

Comments:_____

_____

_____

_____

_____

_____

One Word   Success Score (1-10)

DAY 35
WEEK 5

DATE __/__/__

1 - 10 SCORE

Energy:	"Big M":	Health:	Mood:	Stress:

DIET   Success Score:_____

Meals:_____

_____

_____

_____

_____

DATA

Weight:	Fat %:	x1: _____	x2: _____

MACRONUTRIENT CALCULATIONS

Carbs:	Protein:	Fat:	Calories:

_____

_____

_____

_____

Snacks:_____

_____

Comments:_____

_____

_____

_____

PRIMAL LIFESTYLE   Success Score:_____

Sleep (1-10):_____   Comments:_____
Sun (1-10):_____   Comments:_____
Play (1-10):_____   Comments:_____
Brain (1-10):_____   Comments:_____
Move (1-10):_____   Comments:_____

PERSONAL

Comments:_____

_____

_____

_____

EXERCISE

Success Score:_____   Effort Score:_____

Workout:_____

Location:_____ Duration:_____

Exercise 1:_____Weight:_____ Reps/Time:_____ Set 2:_____ Set 3:_____

Exercise 2:_____Weight:_____ Reps/Time:_____ Set 2:_____ Set 3:_____

Exercise 3:_____Weight:_____ Reps/Time:_____ Set 2:_____ Set 3:_____

Exercise 4:_____Weight:_____ Reps/Time:_____ Set 2:_____ Set 3:_____

Exercise 5:_____Weight:_____ Reps/Time:_____ Set 2:_____ Set 3:_____

Exercise 6:_____Weight:_____ Reps/Time:_____ Set 2:_____ Set 3:_____

Comments:_____

_____

_____

_____

_____

Workout:_____

Location:_____ Distance:_____ Duration:_____

Comments:_____

_____

_____

_____

_____

SUMMARY

Tomorrow:_____

This Week:_____ This Month:_____

Wins:_____

Challenges:_____

Comments:_____

_____

_____

_____   ┌──────────┐ ┌──────────┐

_____   │   │ │   │

_____   └──────────┘ └──────────┘

One Word   Success Score (1-10)

DAY 36
WEEK 6

DATE

/ /

1 - 10 SCORE

Energy:	"Big M":	Health:	Mood:	Stress:

DIET

Success Score:_____

DATA

Weight:	Fat %:	x1: _____	x2: _____

Meals:_____

_____

MACRONUTRIENT CALCULATIONS

Carbs:	Protein:	Fat:	Calories:

_____

_____

_____

_____

_____

_____

Snacks:_____

_____

Comments:_____

_____

_____

_____

PRIMAL LIFESTYLE

Success Score:_____

Sleep (1-10):_____ Comments:_____

Sun (1-10):_____ Comments:_____

Play (1-10):_____ Comments:_____

Brain (1-10):_____ Comments:_____

Move (1-10):_____ Comments:_____

PERSONAL

Comments:_____

_____

_____

_____

EXERCISE   Success Score:_____   Effort Score:_____

Workout:_____

Location:_____ Duration:_____

Exercise 1:_____ Weight:_____ Reps/Time:_____ Set 2:_____ Set 3:_____

Exercise 2:_____ Weight:_____ Reps/Time:_____ Set 2:_____ Set 3:_____

Exercise 3:_____ Weight:_____ Reps/Time:_____ Set 2:_____ Set 3:_____

Exercise 4:_____ Weight:_____ Reps/Time:_____ Set 2:_____ Set 3:_____

Exercise 5:_____ Weight:_____ Reps/Time:_____ Set 2:_____ Set 3:_____

Exercise 6:_____ Weight:_____ Reps/Time:_____ Set 2:_____ Set 3:_____

Comments:_____

_____

_____

_____

_____

Workout:_____

Location:_____ Distance:_____ Duration:_____

Comments:_____

_____

_____

_____

SUMMARY

Tomorrow:_____

This Week:_____ This Month:_____

Wins:_____

Challenges:_____

Comments:_____

_____

_____

_____

_____

_____

One Word   Success Score (1-10)

DAY 37
WEEK 6

DATE ___/___/___

1 - 10 SCORE

Energy:	"Big M":	Health:	Mood:	Stress:

DIET

Success Score:_____

Meals:_____

_____

_____

_____

_____

DATA

Weight:	Fat %:	x1: _____	x2: _____

MACRONUTRIENT CALCULATIONS

Carbs:	Protein:	Fat:	Calories:

_____

_____

_____

_____

Snacks:_____

_____

Comments:_____

_____

_____

_____

PRIMAL LIFESTYLE

Success Score:_____

Sleep (1-10):_____ Comments:_____

Sun (1-10):_____ Comments:_____

Play (1-10):_____ Comments:_____

Brain (1-10):_____ Comments:_____

Move (1-10):_____ Comments:_____

PERSONAL

Comments:_____

_____

_____

_____

EXERCISE Success Score:_____ Effort Score:_____

Workout:_____

Location:_____ Duration:_____

Exercise 1:_____ Weight:_____ Reps/Time:_____ Set 2:_____ Set 3:_____

Exercise 2:_____ Weight:_____ Reps/Time:_____ Set 2:_____ Set 3:_____

Exercise 3:_____ Weight:_____ Reps/Time:_____ Set 2:_____ Set 3:_____

Exercise 4:_____ Weight:_____ Reps/Time:_____ Set 2:_____ Set 3:_____

Exercise 5:_____ Weight:_____ Reps/Time:_____ Set 2:_____ Set 3:_____

Exercise 6:_____ Weight:_____ Reps/Time:_____ Set 2:_____ Set 3:_____

Comments:_____

_____

_____

_____

_____

Workout:_____

Location:_____ Distance:_____ Duration:_____

Comments:_____

_____

_____

_____

_____

SUMMARY

Tomorrow:_____

This Week:_____ This Month:_____

Wins:_____

Challenges:_____

Comments:_____

_____

_____

_____

_____

_____

One Word   Success Score (1-10)

DAY 38
WEEK 6

DATE / /

1 - 10 SCORE

Energy:	"Big M":	Health:	Mood:	Stress:

DIET

Success Score:_____

Meals:_____

_____

_____

_____

DATA

Weight:	Fat %:	x1: _____	x2: _____

MACRONUTRIENT CALCULATIONS

Carbs:	Protein:	Fat:	Calories:

_____

_____

_____

_____

Snacks:_____

_____

Comments:_____

_____

_____

_____

PRIMAL LIFESTYLE

Success Score:_____

Sleep (1-10):_____ Comments:_____

Sun (1-10):_____ Comments:_____

Play (1-10):_____ Comments:_____

Brain (1-10):_____ Comments:_____

Move (1-10):_____ Comments:_____

PERSONAL

Comments:_____

_____

_____

_____

EXERCISE

Success Score:_____ Effort Score:_____

Workout:_____

Location:_____ Duration:_____

Exercise 1:_____ Weight:_____ Reps/Time:_____ Set 2:_____ Set 3:_____

Exercise 2:_____ Weight:_____ Reps/Time:_____ Set 2:_____ Set 3:_____

Exercise 3:_____ Weight:_____ Reps/Time:_____ Set 2:_____ Set 3:_____

Exercise 4:_____ Weight:_____ Reps/Time:_____ Set 2:_____ Set 3:_____

Exercise 5:_____ Weight:_____ Reps/Time:_____ Set 2:_____ Set 3:_____

Exercise 6:_____ Weight:_____ Reps/Time:_____ Set 2:_____ Set 3:_____

Comments:_____

_____

_____

_____

_____

Workout:_____

Location:_____ Distance:_____ Duration:_____

Comments:_____

_____

_____

_____

SUMMARY

Tomorrow:_____

This Week:_____ This Month:_____

Wins:_____

Challenges:_____

Comments:_____

_____

_____

_____

_____

_____

| One Word | Success Score (1-10) |

DAY 39
WEEK 6

DATE
/ /

1 - 10 SCORE

Energy:	"Big M":	Health:	Mood:	Stress:

DIET   Success Score:_____

DATA

Weight:	Fat %:	x1: _____	x2: _____

Meals:_____

MACRONUTRIENT CALCULATIONS

Carbs:	Protein:	Fat:	Calories:

_____

_____

_____

_____

_____

_____

_____

Snacks:_____

Comments:_____

_____

_____

_____

PRIMAL LIFESTYLE   Success Score:_____

Sleep (1-10):_____ Comments:_____

Sun (1-10):_____ Comments:_____

Play (1-10):_____ Comments:_____

Brain (1-10):_____ Comments:_____

Move (1-10):_____ Comments:_____

PERSONAL

Comments:_____

_____

_____

_____

EXERCISE

Success Score:_____   Effort Score:_____

Workout:_____

Location:_____ Duration:_____

Exercise 1:_____Weight:_____Reps/Time:_____Set 2:_____Set 3:_____

Exercise 2:_____Weight:_____Reps/Time:_____Set 2:_____Set 3:_____

Exercise 3:_____Weight:_____Reps/Time:_____Set 2:_____Set 3:_____

Exercise 4:_____Weight:_____Reps/Time:_____Set 2:_____Set 3:_____

Exercise 5:_____Weight:_____Reps/Time:_____Set 2:_____Set 3:_____

Exercise 6:_____Weight:_____Reps/Time:_____Set 2:_____Set 3:_____

Comments:_____

_____

_____

_____

_____

Workout:_____

Location:_____ Distance:_____ Duration:_____

Comments:_____

_____

_____

_____

_____

SUMMARY

Tomorrow:_____

This Week:_____ This Month:_____

Wins:_____

Challenges:_____

Comments:_____

_____

_____

_____

One Word   Success Score (1-10)

DAY 40
WEEK 6

DATE ___/___/___

1 - 10 SCORE

Energy:	"Big M":	Health:	Mood:	Stress:

DIET   Success Score:_____

Meals:_____

_____

_____

_____

DATA

Weight:	Fat %:	x1: _____	x2: _____

MACRONUTRIENT CALCULATIONS

Carbs:	Protein:	Fat:	Calories:

_____

_____

_____

_____

Snacks:_____

_____

Comments:_____

_____

_____

_____

PRIMAL LIFESTYLE   Success Score:_____

Sleep (1-10):_____   Comments:_____

Sun (1-10):_____   Comments:_____

Play (1-10):_____   Comments:_____

Brain (1-10):_____   Comments:_____

Move (1-10):_____   Comments:_____

PERSONAL

Comments:_____

_____

_____

_____

EXERCISE   Success Score:_____   Effort Score:_____

Workout:_____

Location:_____ Duration:_____

Exercise 1:	Weight:	Reps/Time:	Set 2:	Set 3:
Exercise 2:	Weight:	Reps/Time:	Set 2:	Set 3:
Exercise 3:	Weight:	Reps/Time:	Set 2:	Set 3:
Exercise 4:	Weight:	Reps/Time:	Set 2:	Set 3:
Exercise 5:	Weight:	Reps/Time:	Set 2:	Set 3:
Exercise 6:	Weight:	Reps/Time:	Set 2:	Set 3:

Comments:_____

_____

_____

_____

_____

Workout:_____

Location:_____ Distance:_____ Duration:_____

Comments:_____

_____

_____

_____

SUMMARY

Tomorrow:_____

This Week:_____ This Month:_____

Wins:_____

Challenges:_____

Comments:_____

_____

_____

_____

_____

_____

One Word   Success Score (1-10)

DAY 41
WEEK 6

DATE

/ /

1 - 10 SCORE

Energy:	"Big M":	Health:	Mood:	Stress:

DIET   Success Score:_____

DATA

Weight:	Fat %:	x1: _____	x2: _____

Meals:_____

MACRONUTRIENT CALCULATIONS

Carbs:	Protein:	Fat:	Calories:

_____

_____

_____

_____

_____

_____

_____

_____

Snacks:_____

_____

Comments:_____

_____

_____

_____

PRIMAL LIFESTYLE   Success Score:_____

Sleep (1-10):_____   Comments:_____

Sun (1-10):_____   Comments:_____

Play (1-10):_____   Comments:_____

Brain (1-10):_____   Comments:_____

Move (1-10):_____   Comments:_____

PERSONAL

Comments:_____

_____

_____

_____

EXERCISE   Success Score:_____   Effort Score:_____

Workout:_____

Location:_____ Duration:_____

Exercise 1:_____ Weight:_____ Reps/Time:_____ Set 2:_____ Set 3:_____

Exercise 2:_____ Weight:_____ Reps/Time:_____ Set 2:_____ Set 3:_____

Exercise 3:_____ Weight:_____ Reps/Time:_____ Set 2:_____ Set 3:_____

Exercise 4:_____ Weight:_____ Reps/Time:_____ Set 2:_____ Set 3:_____

Exercise 5:_____ Weight:_____ Reps/Time:_____ Set 2:_____ Set 3:_____

Exercise 6:_____ Weight:_____ Reps/Time:_____ Set 2:_____ Set 3:_____

Comments:_____

_____

_____

_____

_____

Workout:_____

Location:_____ Distance:_____ Duration:_____

Comments:_____

_____

_____

_____

SUMMARY

Tomorrow:_____

This Week:_____ This Month:_____

Wins:_____

Challenges:_____

Comments:_____

_____

_____

_____

_____

One Word   Success Score (1-10)

DAY 42
WEEK 6

DATE __ / __ / __

1 - 10 SCORE

Energy:	"Big M":	Health:	Mood:	Stress:

DIET   Success Score:_____

Meals:_____

_____

_____

_____

DATA

Weight:	Fat %:	x1: _____	x2: _____

MACRONUTRIENT CALCULATIONS

Carbs:	Protein:	Fat:	Calories:

_____

_____

_____

_____

Snacks:_____

Comments:_____

_____

_____

_____

PRIMAL LIFESTYLE   Success Score:_____

Sleep (1-10):_____   Comments:_____

Sun (1-10):_____   Comments:_____

Play (1-10):_____   Comments:_____

Brain (1-10):_____   Comments:_____

Move (1-10):_____   Comments:_____

PERSONAL

Comments:_____

_____

_____

_____

EXERCISE   Success Score:_____   Effort Score:_____

Workout:_____

Location:_____ Duration:_____

Exercise 1:_____ Weight:_____ Reps/Time:_____ Set 2:_____ Set 3:_____

Exercise 2:_____ Weight:_____ Reps/Time:_____ Set 2:_____ Set 3:_____

Exercise 3:_____ Weight:_____ Reps/Time:_____ Set 2:_____ Set 3:_____

Exercise 4:_____ Weight:_____ Reps/Time:_____ Set 2:_____ Set 3:_____

Exercise 5:_____ Weight:_____ Reps/Time:_____ Set 2:_____ Set 3:_____

Exercise 6:_____ Weight:_____ Reps/Time:_____ Set 2:_____ Set 3:_____

Comments:_____

_____

_____

_____

_____

Workout:_____

Location:_____ Distance:_____ Duration:_____

Comments:_____

_____

_____

_____

_____

SUMMARY

Tomorrow:_____

This Week:_____ This Month:_____

Wins:_____

Challenges:_____

Comments:_____

_____

_____

_____

_____

One Word   Success Score (1-10)

DAY 43
WEEK 7

DATE / /

Energy:	"Big M":	Health:	Mood:	Stress:

DIET

Success Score:_____

Meals:_____

_____

_____

_____

_____

DATA

Weight:	Fat %:	x1: _____	x2: _____

MACRONUTRIENT CALCULATIONS

Carbs:	Protein:	Fat:	Calories:

_____

_____

_____

_____

Snacks:_____

_____

Comments:_____

_____

_____

_____

PRIMAL LIFESTYLE

Success Score:_____

Sleep (1-10):_____ Comments:_____

Sun (1-10):_____ Comments:_____

Play (1-10):_____ Comments:_____

Brain (1-10):_____ Comments:_____

Move (1-10):_____ Comments:_____

PERSONAL

Comments:_____

_____

_____

_____

EXERCISE   Success Score:_____   Effort Score:_____

Workout:_____

Location:_____ Duration:_____

Exercise 1:_____ Weight:_____ Reps/Time:_____ Set 2:_____ Set 3:_____

Exercise 2:_____ Weight:_____ Reps/Time:_____ Set 2:_____ Set 3:_____

Exercise 3:_____ Weight:_____ Reps/Time:_____ Set 2:_____ Set 3:_____

Exercise 4:_____ Weight:_____ Reps/Time:_____ Set 2:_____ Set 3:_____

Exercise 5:_____ Weight:_____ Reps/Time:_____ Set 2:_____ Set 3:_____

Exercise 6:_____ Weight:_____ Reps/Time:_____ Set 2:_____ Set 3:_____

Comments:_____

_____

_____

_____

_____

Workout:_____

Location:_____ Distance:_____ Duration:_____

Comments:_____

_____

_____

_____

SUMMARY

Tomorrow:_____

This Week:_____ This Month:_____

Wins:_____

Challenges:_____

Comments:_____

_____

_____

_____

_____

_____

One Word   Success Score (1-10)

DAY 44
WEEK 7

DATE / /

1 - 10 SCORE

Energy:	"Big M":	Health:	Mood:	Stress:

DIET

Success Score:_____

Meals:_____

_____

_____

_____

DATA

Weight:	Fat %:	x1: _____	x2: _____

MACRONUTRIENT CALCULATIONS

Carbs:	Protein:	Fat:	Calories:

_____

_____

_____

_____

Snacks:_____

_____

Comments:_____

_____

_____

_____

PRIMAL LIFESTYLE

Success Score:_____

Sleep (1-10):_____ Comments:_____

Sun (1-10):_____ Comments:_____

Play (1-10):_____ Comments:_____

Brain (1-10):_____ Comments:_____

Move (1-10):_____ Comments:_____

PERSONAL

Comments:_____

_____

_____

_____

EXERCISE   Success Score:_____ Effort Score:_____

Workout:_____

Location:_____ Duration:_____

Exercise 1:_____Weight:_____Reps/Time:_____Set 2:_____Set 3:_____

Exercise 2:_____Weight:_____Reps/Time:_____Set 2:_____Set 3:_____

Exercise 3:_____Weight:_____Reps/Time:_____Set 2:_____Set 3:_____

Exercise 4:_____Weight:_____Reps/Time:_____Set 2:_____Set 3:_____

Exercise 5:_____Weight:_____Reps/Time:_____Set 2:_____Set 3:_____

Exercise 6:_____Weight:_____Reps/Time:_____Set 2:_____Set 3:_____

Comments:_____

_____

_____

_____

_____

Workout:_____

Location:_____ Distance:_____ Duration:_____

Comments:_____

_____

_____

_____

SUMMARY

Tomorrow:_____

This Week:_____ This Month:_____

Wins:_____

Challenges:_____

Comments:_____

_____

_____

_____

_____

_____

One Word   Success Score (1-10)

DAY 45
WEEK 7

DATE __ / __ / __

1 - 10 SCORE

Energy:	"Big M":	Health:	Mood:	Stress:

DIET   Success Score:_____

Meals:_____

_____

_____

_____

_____

DATA

Weight:	Fat %:	x1: _____	x2: _____

MACRONUTRIENT CALCULATIONS

Carbs:	Protein:	Fat:	Calories:

_____

_____

_____

_____

Snacks:_____

Comments:_____

_____

_____

_____

PRIMAL LIFESTYLE   Success Score:_____

Sleep (1-10):_____ Comments:_____

Sun (1-10):_____ Comments:_____

Play (1-10):_____ Comments:_____

Brain (1-10):_____ Comments:_____

Move (1-10):_____ Comments:_____

PERSONAL

Comments:_____

_____

_____

_____

EXERCISE   Success Score:_____   Effort Score:_____

Workout:_____

Location:_____ Duration:_____

Exercise 1:_____ Weight:_____ Reps/Time:_____ Set 2:_____ Set 3:_____

Exercise 2:_____ Weight:_____ Reps/Time:_____ Set 2:_____ Set 3:_____

Exercise 3:_____ Weight:_____ Reps/Time:_____ Set 2:_____ Set 3:_____

Exercise 4:_____ Weight:_____ Reps/Time:_____ Set 2:_____ Set 3:_____

Exercise 5:_____ Weight:_____ Reps/Time:_____ Set 2:_____ Set 3:_____

Exercise 6:_____ Weight:_____ Reps/Time:_____ Set 2:_____ Set 3:_____

Comments:_____

_____

_____

_____

_____

Workout:_____

Location:_____ Distance:_____ Duration:_____

Comments:_____

_____

_____

_____

SUMMARY

Tomorrow:_____

This Week:_____ This Month:_____

Wins:_____

Challenges:_____

Comments:_____

_____

_____

_____

One Word   Success Score (1-10)

DAY 46
WEEK 7

DATE _/_ /_

1 - 10 SCORE

Energy:	"Big M":	Health:	Mood:	Stress:

DIET   Success Score:_____

Meals:_____

_____

_____

_____

_____

DATA

Weight:	Fat %:	x1: _____	x2: _____

MACRONUTRIENT CALCULATIONS

Carbs:	Protein:	Fat:	Calories:

_____

_____

_____

_____

Snacks:_____

_____

Comments:_____

_____

_____

_____

PRIMAL LIFESTYLE   Success Score:_____

Sleep (1-10):_____   Comments:_____

Sun (1-10):_____   Comments:_____

Play (1-10):_____   Comments:_____

Brain (1-10):_____   Comments:_____

Move (1-10):_____   Comments:_____

PERSONAL

Comments:_____

_____

_____

_____

EXERCISE   Success Score:_____   Effort Score:_____

Workout:_____

Location:_____ Duration:_____

Exercise 1:_____ Weight:_____ Reps/Time:_____ Set 2:_____ Set 3:_____

Exercise 2:_____ Weight:_____ Reps/Time:_____ Set 2:_____ Set 3:_____

Exercise 3:_____ Weight:_____ Reps/Time:_____ Set 2:_____ Set 3:_____

Exercise 4:_____ Weight:_____ Reps/Time:_____ Set 2:_____ Set 3:_____

Exercise 5:_____ Weight:_____ Reps/Time:_____ Set 2:_____ Set 3:_____

Exercise 6:_____ Weight:_____ Reps/Time:_____ Set 2:_____ Set 3:_____

Comments:_____

_____

_____

_____

_____

Workout:_____

Location:_____ Distance:_____ Duration:_____

Comments:_____

_____

_____

_____

SUMMARY

Tomorrow:_____

This Week:_____ This Month:_____

Wins:_____

Challenges:_____

Comments:_____

_____

_____

_____   _____ _____

_____

_____   One Word   Success Score (1-10)

DAY 47
WEEK 7

DATE ___/___/___

DIET   Success Score:_____

DATA

Weight:	Fat %:	x1: _____	x2: _____

Meals:_____

MACRONUTRIENT CALCULATIONS

Carbs:	Protein:	Fat:	Calories:

_____

_____

_____

_____

_____

_____

_____

_____

Snacks:_____

_____

Comments:_____

_____

_____

_____

PRIMAL LIFESTYLE   Success Score:_____

Sleep (1-10):_____   Comments:_____

Sun (1-10):_____   Comments:_____

Play (1-10):_____   Comments:_____

Brain (1-10):_____   Comments:_____

Move (1-10):_____   Comments:_____

PERSONAL

Comments:_____

_____

_____

_____

EXERCISE   Success Score:_____   Effort Score:_____

Workout:_____

Location:_____ Duration:_____

Exercise 1:_____Weight:_____Reps/Time:_____Set 2:_____Set 3:_____

Exercise 2:_____Weight:_____Reps/Time:_____Set 2:_____Set 3:_____

Exercise 3:_____Weight:_____Reps/Time:_____Set 2:_____Set 3:_____

Exercise 4:_____Weight:_____Reps/Time:_____Set 2:_____Set 3:_____

Exercise 5:_____Weight:_____Reps/Time:_____Set 2:_____Set 3:_____

Exercise 6:_____Weight:_____Reps/Time:_____Set 2:_____Set 3:_____

Comments:_____

_____

_____

_____

_____

Workout:_____

Location:_____ Distance:_____ Duration:_____

Comments:_____

_____

_____

_____

SUMMARY

Tomorrow:_____

This Week:_____ This Month:_____

Wins:_____

Challenges:_____

Comments:_____

_____

_____

_____

One Word   Success Score (1-10)

DAY 48
WEEK 7

DATE ___/___/___

1 - 10 SCORE

Energy:	"Big M":	Health:	Mood:	Stress:

DIET

Success Score:_____

Meals:_____

_____

_____

_____

DATA

Weight:	Fat %:	x1: _____	x2: _____

MACRONUTRIENT CALCULATIONS

Carbs:	Protein:	Fat:	Calories:

_____

_____

_____

_____

Snacks:_____

Comments:_____

_____

_____

_____

PRIMAL LIFESTYLE

Success Score:_____

Sleep (1-10):_____ Comments:_____

Sun (1-10):_____ Comments:_____

Play (1-10):_____ Comments:_____

Brain (1-10):_____ Comments:_____

Move (1-10):_____ Comments:_____

PERSONAL

Comments:_____

_____

_____

_____

EXERCISE   Success Score:_____   Effort Score:_____

Workout:_____

Location:_____   Duration:_____

Exercise 1:_____	Weight:_____	Reps/Time:_____	Set 2:_____	Set 3:_____
Exercise 2:_____	Weight:_____	Reps/Time:_____	Set 2:_____	Set 3:_____
Exercise 3:_____	Weight:_____	Reps/Time:_____	Set 2:_____	Set 3:_____
Exercise 4:_____	Weight:_____	Reps/Time:_____	Set 2:_____	Set 3:_____
Exercise 5:_____	Weight:_____	Reps/Time:_____	Set 2:_____	Set 3:_____
Exercise 6:_____	Weight:_____	Reps/Time:_____	Set 2:_____	Set 3:_____

Comments:_____
_____
_____
_____
_____

Workout:_____

Location:_____   Distance:_____   Duration:_____

Comments:_____
_____
_____
_____

SUMMARY

Tomorrow:_____

This Week:_____   This Month:_____

Wins:_____

Challenges:_____

Comments:_____
_____
_____
_____

_____

_____

One Word   Success Score (1-10)

DAY 49
WEEK 7

DATE
/ /

1 - 10 SCORE

Energy:	"Big M":	Health:	Mood:	Stress:

DIET   Success Score:_____

Meals:_____

_____

_____

_____

_____

DATA

Weight:	Fat %:	x1: _____	x2: _____

MACRONUTRIENT CALCULATIONS

Carbs:	Protein:	Fat:	Calories:

_____

_____

_____

_____

Snacks:_____

_____

Comments:_____

_____

_____

_____

PRIMAL LIFESTYLE   Success Score:_____

Sleep (1-10):_____ Comments:_____
Sun (1-10):_____ Comments:_____
Play (1-10):_____ Comments:_____
Brain (1-10):_____ Comments:_____
Move (1-10):_____ Comments:_____

PERSONAL

Comments:_____

_____

_____

_____

EXERCISE   Success Score:_____   Effort Score:_____

Workout:_____

Location:_____ Duration:_____

Exercise 1:_____ Weight:_____ Reps/Time:_____ Set 2:_____ Set 3:_____

Exercise 2:_____ Weight:_____ Reps/Time:_____ Set 2:_____ Set 3:_____

Exercise 3:_____ Weight:_____ Reps/Time:_____ Set 2:_____ Set 3:_____

Exercise 4:_____ Weight:_____ Reps/Time:_____ Set 2:_____ Set 3:_____

Exercise 5:_____ Weight:_____ Reps/Time:_____ Set 2:_____ Set 3:_____

Exercise 6:_____ Weight:_____ Reps/Time:_____ Set 2:_____ Set 3:_____

Comments:_____

_____

_____

_____

_____

Workout:_____

Location:_____ Distance:_____ Duration:_____

Comments:_____

_____

_____

_____

SUMMARY

Tomorrow:_____

This Week:_____ This Month:_____

Wins:_____

Challenges:_____

Comments:_____

_____

_____

_____

_____

_____

One Word   Success Score (1-10)

DAY 50
WEEK 8

DATE ___/___/___

1 - 10 SCORE

Energy:	"Big M":	Health:	Mood:	Stress:

DIET   Success Score:_____

Meals:_____

_____

_____

_____

_____

DATA

Weight:	Fat %:	x1: _____	x2: _____

MACRONUTRIENT CALCULATIONS

Carbs:	Protein:	Fat:	Calories:

_____

_____

_____

_____

Snacks:_____

_____

Comments:_____

_____

_____

_____

PRIMAL LIFESTYLE   Success Score:_____

Sleep (1-10):_____ Comments:_____

Sun (1-10):_____ Comments:_____

Play (1-10):_____ Comments:_____

Brain (1-10):_____ Comments:_____

Move (1-10):_____ Comments:_____

PERSONAL

Comments:_____

_____

_____

_____

EXERCISE   Success Score:_____   Effort Score:_____

Workout:_____

Location:_____ Duration:_____

Exercise 1:_____Weight:_____Reps/Time:_____Set 2:_____Set 3:_____
Exercise 2:_____Weight:_____Reps/Time:_____Set 2:_____Set 3:_____
Exercise 3:_____Weight:_____Reps/Time:_____Set 2:_____Set 3:_____
Exercise 4:_____Weight:_____Reps/Time:_____Set 2:_____Set 3:_____
Exercise 5:_____Weight:_____Reps/Time:_____Set 2:_____Set 3:_____
Exercise 6:_____Weight:_____Reps/Time:_____Set 2:_____Set 3:_____

Comments:_____
_____
_____
_____
_____

Workout:_____

Location:_____ Distance:_____ Duration:_____

Comments:_____
_____
_____
_____

SUMMARY

Tomorrow:_____

This Week:_____ This Month:_____

Wins:_____

Challenges:_____

Comments:_____
_____
_____
_____
_____
_____

One Word   Success Score (1-10)

DAY 51
WEEK 8

DATE / /

1 - 10 SCORE

Energy:	"Big M":	Health:	Mood:	Stress:

DIET   Success Score:_____

Meals:_____

_____

_____

_____

_____

DATA

Weight:	Fat %:	x1: _____	x2: _____

MACRONUTRIENT CALCULATIONS

Carbs:	Protein:	Fat:	Calories:

_____

_____

_____

_____

Snacks:_____

_____

Comments:_____

_____

_____

_____

PRIMAL LIFESTYLE   Success Score:_____

Sleep (1-10):_____   Comments:_____

Sun (1-10):_____   Comments:_____

Play (1-10):_____   Comments:_____

Brain (1-10):_____   Comments:_____

Move (1-10):_____   Comments:_____

PERSONAL

Comments:_____

_____

_____

_____

EXERCISE   Success Score:_____   Effort Score:_____

Workout:_____

Location:_____   Duration:_____

Exercise 1:_____ Weight:_____ Reps/Time:_____ Set 2:_____ Set 3:_____

Exercise 2:_____ Weight:_____ Reps/Time:_____ Set 2:_____ Set 3:_____

Exercise 3:_____ Weight:_____ Reps/Time:_____ Set 2:_____ Set 3:_____

Exercise 4:_____ Weight:_____ Reps/Time:_____ Set 2:_____ Set 3:_____

Exercise 5:_____ Weight:_____ Reps/Time:_____ Set 2:_____ Set 3:_____

Exercise 6:_____ Weight:_____ Reps/Time:_____ Set 2:_____ Set 3:_____

Comments:_____

_____

_____

_____

_____

Workout:_____

Location:_____ Distance:_____ Duration:_____

Comments:_____

_____

_____

_____

SUMMARY

Tomorrow:_____

This Week:_____ This Month:_____

Wins:_____

Challenges:_____

Comments:_____

_____

_____

_____   _____

One Word   Success Score (1-10)

DAY 52
WEEK 8

DATE __/__/__

1 - 10 SCORE

Energy:	"Big M":	Health:	Mood:	Stress:

DIET   Success Score:_____

DATA

Weight:	Fat %:	x1: _____	x2: _____

Meals:_____

_____

_____

MACRONUTRIENT CALCULATIONS

Carbs:	Protein:	Fat:	Calories:

_____

_____

_____

_____

_____

_____

_____

Snacks:_____

_____

Comments:_____

_____

_____

_____

PRIMAL LIFESTYLE   Success Score:_____

Sleep (1-10):_____   Comments:_____

Sun (1-10):_____   Comments:_____

Play (1-10):_____   Comments:_____

Brain (1-10):_____   Comments:_____

Move (1-10):_____   Comments:_____

PERSONAL

Comments:_____

_____

_____

_____

EXERCISE   Success Score:_____   Effort Score:_____

Workout:_____

Location:_____ Duration:_____

Exercise 1:_____ Weight:_____ Reps/Time:_____ Set 2:_____ Set 3:_____

Exercise 2:_____ Weight:_____ Reps/Time:_____ Set 2:_____ Set 3:_____

Exercise 3:_____ Weight:_____ Reps/Time:_____ Set 2:_____ Set 3:_____

Exercise 4:_____ Weight:_____ Reps/Time:_____ Set 2:_____ Set 3:_____

Exercise 5:_____ Weight:_____ Reps/Time:_____ Set 2:_____ Set 3:_____

Exercise 6:_____ Weight:_____ Reps/Time:_____ Set 2:_____ Set 3:_____

Comments:_____

_____

_____

_____

_____

Workout:_____

Location:_____ Distance:_____ Duration:_____

Comments:_____

_____

_____

_____

SUMMARY

Tomorrow:_____

This Week:_____ This Month:_____

Wins:_____

Challenges:_____

Comments:_____

_____

_____

_____

_____

One Word   Success Score (1-10)

DAY 53
WEEK 8

DATE / /

1 - 10 SCORE

Energy:	"Big M":	Health:	Mood:	Stress:

DIET

Success Score:_____

Meals:_____

_____

_____

_____

_____

DATA

Weight:	Fat %:	x1: _____	x2: _____

MACRONUTRIENT CALCULATIONS

Carbs:	Protein:	Fat:	Calories:

_____

_____

_____

_____

Snacks:_____

Comments:_____

_____

_____

_____

PRIMAL LIFESTYLE

Success Score:_____

Sleep (1-10):_____ Comments:_____

Sun (1-10):_____ Comments:_____

Play (1-10):_____ Comments:_____

Brain (1-10):_____ Comments:_____

Move (1-10):_____ Comments:_____

PERSONAL

Comments:_____

_____

_____

_____

EXERCISE   Success Score:_____   Effort Score:_____

Workout:_____

Location:_____ Duration:_____

Exercise 1:_____ Weight:_____ Reps/Time:_____ Set 2:_____ Set 3:_____

Exercise 2:_____ Weight:_____ Reps/Time:_____ Set 2:_____ Set 3:_____

Exercise 3:_____ Weight:_____ Reps/Time:_____ Set 2:_____ Set 3:_____

Exercise 4:_____ Weight:_____ Reps/Time:_____ Set 2:_____ Set 3:_____

Exercise 5:_____ Weight:_____ Reps/Time:_____ Set 2:_____ Set 3:_____

Exercise 6:_____ Weight:_____ Reps/Time:_____ Set 2:_____ Set 3:_____

Comments:_____

_____

_____

_____

_____

Workout:_____

Location:_____ Distance:_____ Duration:_____

Comments:_____

_____

_____

_____

SUMMARY

Tomorrow:_____

This Week:_____ This Month:_____

Wins:_____

Challenges:_____

Comments:_____

_____

_____

_____

_____

One Word   Success Score (1-10)

DAY 54
WEEK 8

DATE / /

1 - 10 SCORE

Energy:	"Big M":	Health:	Mood:	Stress:

DIET

Success Score:_____

Meals:_____

_____

_____

_____

_____

DATA

Weight:	Fat %:	x1:_____	x2:_____

MACRONUTRIENT CALCULATIONS

Carbs:	Protein:	Fat:	Calories:

_____

_____

_____

_____

Snacks:_____

_____

Comments:_____

_____

_____

PRIMAL LIFESTYLE

Success Score:_____

Sleep (1-10):_____ Comments:_____

Sun (1-10):_____ Comments:_____

Play (1-10):_____ Comments:_____

Brain (1-10):_____ Comments:_____

Move (1-10):_____ Comments:_____

PERSONAL

Comments:_____

_____

_____

_____

EXERCISE

Success Score:_____ Effort Score:_____

Workout:_____

Location:_____ Duration:_____

Exercise 1:_____Weight:_____Reps/Time:_____Set 2:_____Set 3:_____

Exercise 2:_____Weight:_____Reps/Time:_____Set 2:_____Set 3:_____

Exercise 3:_____Weight:_____Reps/Time:_____Set 2:_____Set 3:_____

Exercise 4:_____Weight:_____Reps/Time:_____Set 2:_____Set 3:_____

Exercise 5:_____Weight:_____Reps/Time:_____Set 2:_____Set 3:_____

Exercise 6:_____Weight:_____Reps/Time:_____Set 2:_____Set 3:_____

Comments:_____

_____

_____

_____

_____

Workout:_____

Location:_____ Distance:_____ Duration:_____

Comments:_____

_____

_____

_____

SUMMARY

Tomorrow:_____

This Week:_____ This Month:_____

Wins:_____

Challenges:_____

Comments:_____

_____

_____

_____

_____

_____

One Word   Success Score (1-10)

DAY 55
WEEK 8

DATE / /

1 - 10 SCORE

Energy:	"Big M":	Health:	Mood:	Stress:

DIET

Success Score:_____

Meals:_____

_____

_____

_____

DATA

Weight:	Fat %:	x1: _____	x2: _____

MACRONUTRIENT CALCULATIONS

Carbs:	Protein:	Fat:	Calories:

_____

_____

_____

_____

Snacks:_____

_____

Comments:_____

_____

_____

_____

PRIMAL LIFESTYLE

Success Score:_____

Sleep (1-10):_____ Comments:_____

Sun (1-10):_____ Comments:_____

Play (1-10):_____ Comments:_____

Brain (1-10):_____ Comments:_____

Move (1-10):_____ Comments:_____

PERSONAL

Comments:_____

_____

_____

_____

EXERCISE   Success Score:_____   Effort Score:_____

Workout:_____

Location:_____ Duration:_____

Exercise 1:_____ Weight:_____ Reps/Time:_____ Set 2:_____ Set 3:_____

Exercise 2:_____ Weight:_____ Reps/Time:_____ Set 2:_____ Set 3:_____

Exercise 3:_____ Weight:_____ Reps/Time:_____ Set 2:_____ Set 3:_____

Exercise 4:_____ Weight:_____ Reps/Time:_____ Set 2:_____ Set 3:_____

Exercise 5:_____ Weight:_____ Reps/Time:_____ Set 2:_____ Set 3:_____

Exercise 6:_____ Weight:_____ Reps/Time:_____ Set 2:_____ Set 3:_____

Comments:_____

_____

_____

_____

_____

Workout:_____

Location:_____ Distance:_____ Duration:_____

Comments:_____

_____

_____

_____

SUMMARY

Tomorrow:_____

This Week:_____ This Month:_____

Wins:_____

Challenges:_____

Comments:_____

_____

_____

_____

_____

_____

One Word   Success Score (1-10)

DAY 56
WEEK 8

DATE ___/___/___

1 - 10 SCORE

Energy:	"Big M":	Health:	Mood:	Stress:

DIET   Success Score:_____

Meals:_____

_____

DATA

Weight:	Fat %:	x1: _____	x2: _____

MACRONUTRIENT CALCULATIONS

Carbs:	Protein:	Fat:	Calories:

_____

_____

_____

_____

Snacks:_____

_____

Comments:_____

_____

_____

_____

PRIMAL LIFESTYLE   Success Score:_____

Sleep (1-10):_____   Comments:_____
Sun (1-10):_____   Comments:_____
Play (1-10):_____   Comments:_____
Brain (1-10):_____   Comments:_____
Move (1-10):_____   Comments:_____

PERSONAL

Comments:_____

_____

_____

_____

EXERCISE   Success Score:_____   Effort Score:_____

Workout:_____

Location:_____ Duration:_____

Exercise 1:_____ Weight:_____ Reps/Time:_____ Set 2:_____ Set 3:_____

Exercise 2:_____ Weight:_____ Reps/Time:_____ Set 2:_____ Set 3:_____

Exercise 3:_____ Weight:_____ Reps/Time:_____ Set 2:_____ Set 3:_____

Exercise 4:_____ Weight:_____ Reps/Time:_____ Set 2:_____ Set 3:_____

Exercise 5:_____ Weight:_____ Reps/Time:_____ Set 2:_____ Set 3:_____

Exercise 6:_____ Weight:_____ Reps/Time:_____ Set 2:_____ Set 3:_____

Comments:_____
_____
_____
_____
_____

Workout:_____

Location:_____ Distance:_____ Duration:_____

Comments:_____
_____
_____
_____

SUMMARY

Tomorrow:_____

This Week:_____ This Month:_____

Wins:_____

Challenges:_____

Comments:_____
_____
_____
_____
_____
_____

One Word   Success Score (1-10)

DAY 57
WEEK 9

DATE / /

1 - 10 SCORE

Energy:	"Big M":	Health:	Mood:	Stress:

DIET

Success Score:_____

Meals:_____

_____

_____

_____

_____

DATA

Weight:	Fat %:	x1: _____	x2: _____

MACRONUTRIENT CALCULATIONS

Carbs:	Protein:	Fat:	Calories:

_____

_____

_____

_____

_____

Snacks:_____

_____

Comments:_____

_____

_____

_____

PRIMAL LIFESTYLE

Success Score:_____

Sleep (1-10):_____ Comments:_____

Sun (1-10):_____ Comments:_____

Play (1-10):_____ Comments:_____

Brain (1-10):_____ Comments:_____

Move (1-10):_____ Comments:_____

PERSONAL

Comments:_____

_____

_____

_____

EXERCISE   Success Score:_____   Effort Score:_____

Workout:_____

Location:_____ Duration:_____

Exercise 1:_____ Weight:_____ Reps/Time:_____ Set 2:_____ Set 3:_____

Exercise 2:_____ Weight:_____ Reps/Time:_____ Set 2:_____ Set 3:_____

Exercise 3:_____ Weight:_____ Reps/Time:_____ Set 2:_____ Set 3:_____

Exercise 4:_____ Weight:_____ Reps/Time:_____ Set 2:_____ Set 3:_____

Exercise 5:_____ Weight:_____ Reps/Time:_____ Set 2:_____ Set 3:_____

Exercise 6:_____ Weight:_____ Reps/Time:_____ Set 2:_____ Set 3:_____

Comments:_____

_____

_____

_____

_____

Workout:_____

Location:_____ Distance:_____ Duration:_____

Comments:_____

_____

_____

_____

_____

SUMMARY

Tomorrow:_____

This Week:_____ This Month:_____

Wins:_____

Challenges:_____

Comments:_____

_____

_____

_____

_____

_____

One Word   Success Score (1-10)

DAY 58
WEEK 9

DATE / /

Energy:	"Big M":	Health:	Mood:	Stress:

DIET

Success Score:_____

Meals:_____

_____

_____

_____

DATA

Weight:	Fat %:	x1: _____	x2: _____

MACRONUTRIENT CALCULATIONS

Carbs:	Protein:	Fat:	Calories:

_____

_____

_____

_____

Snacks:_____

_____

Comments:_____

_____

_____

_____

PRIMAL LIFESTYLE

Success Score:_____

Sleep (1-10):_____ Comments:_____

Sun (1-10):_____ Comments:_____

Play (1-10):_____ Comments:_____

Brain (1-10):_____ Comments:_____

Move (1-10):_____ Comments:_____

PERSONAL

Comments:_____

_____

_____

_____

EXERCISE   Success Score:_____   Effort Score:_____

Workout:_____

Location:_____ Duration:_____

Exercise 1:_____ Weight:_____ Reps/Time:_____ Set 2:_____ Set 3:_____

Exercise 2:_____ Weight:_____ Reps/Time:_____ Set 2:_____ Set 3:_____

Exercise 3:_____ Weight:_____ Reps/Time:_____ Set 2:_____ Set 3:_____

Exercise 4:_____ Weight:_____ Reps/Time:_____ Set 2:_____ Set 3:_____

Exercise 5:_____ Weight:_____ Reps/Time:_____ Set 2:_____ Set 3:_____

Exercise 6:_____ Weight:_____ Reps/Time:_____ Set 2:_____ Set 3:_____

Comments:_____

_____

_____

_____

_____

Workout:_____

Location:_____ Distance:_____ Duration:_____

Comments:_____

_____

_____

_____

_____

SUMMARY

Tomorrow:_____

This Week:_____ This Month:_____

Wins:_____

Challenges:_____

Comments:_____

_____

_____

_____

_____

_____

One Word   Success Score (1-10)

DAY 59
WEEK 9

DATE / /

1 - 10 SCORE

Energy:	"Big M":	Health:	Mood:	Stress:

DIET   Success Score:_____

Meals:_____

_____

_____

_____

_____

DATA

Weight:	Fat %:	x1: _____	x2: _____

MACRONUTRIENT CALCULATIONS

Carbs:	Protein:	Fat:	Calories:

_____

_____

_____

_____

Snacks:_____

_____

Comments:_____

_____

_____

_____

PRIMAL LIFESTYLE   Success Score:_____

Sleep (1-10):_____ Comments:_____

Sun (1-10):_____ Comments:_____

Play (1-10):_____ Comments:_____

Brain (1-10):_____ Comments:_____

Move (1-10):_____ Comments:_____

PERSONAL

Comments:_____

_____

_____

_____

EXERCISE   Success Score:_____   Effort Score:_____

Workout:_____
Location:_____ Duration:_____
Exercise 1:_____ Weight:_____ Reps/Time:_____ Set 2:_____ Set 3:_____
Exercise 2:_____ Weight:_____ Reps/Time:_____ Set 2:_____ Set 3:_____
Exercise 3:_____ Weight:_____ Reps/Time:_____ Set 2:_____ Set 3:_____
Exercise 4:_____ Weight:_____ Reps/Time:_____ Set 2:_____ Set 3:_____
Exercise 5:_____ Weight:_____ Reps/Time:_____ Set 2:_____ Set 3:_____
Exercise 6:_____ Weight:_____ Reps/Time:_____ Set 2:_____ Set 3:_____
Comments:_____
_____
_____
_____
_____

Workout:_____
Location:_____ Distance:_____ Duration:_____
Comments:_____
_____
_____
_____
_____

SUMMARY

Tomorrow:_____
This Week:_____ This Month:_____
Wins:_____
Challenges:_____
Comments:_____
_____
_____
_____
_____
_____

One Word   Success Score (1-10)

DAY 60
WEEK 9

1 - 10 SCORE

Energy:	"Big M":	Health:	Mood:	Stress:

DIET   Success Score:_____

Meals:_____

_____

_____

_____

_____

DATA

Weight:	Fat %:	x1: _____	x2: _____

MACRONUTRIENT CALCULATIONS

Carbs:	Protein:	Fat:	Calories:

_____

_____

_____

_____

Snacks:_____

_____

Comments:_____

_____

_____

_____

PRIMAL LIFESTYLE   Success Score:_____

Sleep (1-10):_____ Comments:_____

Sun (1-10):_____ Comments:_____

Play (1-10):_____ Comments:_____

Brain (1-10):_____ Comments:_____

Move (1-10):_____ Comments:_____

PERSONAL

Comments:_____

_____

_____

_____

EXERCISE   Success Score:_____   Effort Score:_____

Workout:_____

Location:_____ Duration:_____

Exercise 1:_____Weight:_____Reps/Time:_____Set 2:_____Set 3:_____

Exercise 2:_____Weight:_____Reps/Time:_____Set 2:_____Set 3:_____

Exercise 3:_____Weight:_____Reps/Time:_____Set 2:_____Set 3:_____

Exercise 4:_____Weight:_____Reps/Time:_____Set 2:_____Set 3:_____

Exercise 5:_____Weight:_____Reps/Time:_____Set 2:_____Set 3:_____

Exercise 6:_____Weight:_____Reps/Time:_____Set 2:_____Set 3:_____

Comments:_____

_____

_____

_____

_____

_____

Workout:_____

Location:_____ Distance:_____ Duration:_____

Comments:_____

_____

_____

_____

_____

SUMMARY

Tomorrow:_____

This Week:_____ This Month:_____

Wins:_____

Challenges:_____

Comments:_____

_____

_____

_____

_____

One Word	Success Score (1-10)

DAY 60 EVALUATION

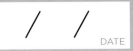 / / DATE

DIET   Past 30 days.

Success Score:_____

Wins:_____

Challenges:_____

Comments:_____

_____

1 - 10 SCORE

Energy:	"Big M":	Health:	Mood:	Stress:

MACRONUTRIENT CALCULATIONS

Carbs:	Protein:	Fat:	Calories:

_____

_____

_____

PRIMAL LIFESTYLE   Past 30 days.

Success Score:_____

Sleep (1-10):_____   Comments:_____

Sun (1-10):_____   Comments:_____

Play (1-10):_____   Comments:_____

Brain (1-10):_____   Comments:_____

Move (1-10):_____   Comments:_____

PERSONAL   Past 30 days.

Comments:_____

_____

_____

_____

_____

_____

_____

_____

DAY 60 EVALUATION

EXERCISE   Past 30 days.

Success Score:_____   Effort Score:_____

Wins:_____

Challenges:_____

Comments:_____

_____

_____

_____

GOALS

1._____

2._____

3._____

4._____

5._____

BODY MEASUREMENTS

Time of Day:_____   Scale/method used:_____

Day 1 weight:_____   Day 1 fat %:_____

Day 2 weight:_____   Day 2 fat %:_____

Day 3 weight:_____   Day 3 fat %:_____

Average weight:_____   Average body fat %:_____

Body part measurements:.

Waistline:_____ Hips:_____ Chest:_____

Thighs:_____ Biceps:_____

Other body measurement:_____ Value:_____

Other body measurement:_____ Value:_____

DAY 60 EVALUATION

FITNESS MEASUREMENTS

Morning resting heart rate:_____   _____   _____   Average:_____
　　　　　　　　　　　　　　　　Day 1　　　　　Day 2　　　　Day 3

Primal Essential Movements – one set maximum effort

Note type of progression or advanced exercise if not actual Essential Movement
(e.g. – decline pushups, chair-assisted pullups)

Pushups:_____   Number:_____

Pullups:_____   Number:_____

Squats:_____   Number:_____

Plank:_____   Time:_____

400 meter run:_____   Date:_____

Location/conditions/notes:_____

One-mile run:_____   Date:_____

Location/conditions/notes:_____

_____

Maximum Aerobic Function test

Date:_____ Heart Rate:_____

Course/distance:_____   Time:_____

Location/conditions/notes:_____

VO2 Max test (ml/kg value):_____

Date/location/method of test:_____

Other best performances:

Event/Exercise:_____   Achievement:_____

Event/Exercise:_____   Achievement:_____

Event/Exercise:_____   Achievement:_____

"What was lacking in my previous weight loss attempts was not self-discipline or motivation, but the conventional approach itself. Some well-intentioned skeptics expressed long-term health concerns over my low-carb Primal eating, but I've learned to let results (lost 150 pounds in 16 months) speak for themselves."

– Success Story Charlie

DAY 61
WEEK 9

DATE / /

1 - 10 SCORE

Energy:	"Big M":	Health:	Mood:	Stress:

DIET   Success Score:_____

Meals:_____

_____

_____

_____

_____

DATA

Weight:	Fat %:	x1: _____	x2: _____

MACRONUTRIENT CALCULATIONS

Carbs:	Protein:	Fat:	Calories:

_____

_____

_____

_____

_____

Snacks:_____

_____

Comments:_____

_____

_____

_____

PRIMAL LIFESTYLE   Success Score:_____

Sleep (1-10):_____   Comments:_____

Sun (1-10):_____   Comments:_____

Play (1-10):_____   Comments:_____

Brain (1-10):_____   Comments:_____

Move (1-10):_____   Comments:_____

PERSONAL

Comments:_____

_____

_____

_____

EXERCISE   Success Score:_____   Effort Score:_____

Workout:_____

Location:_____ Duration:_____

Exercise 1:_____	Weight:_____	Reps/Time:_____	Set 2:_____	Set 3:_____
Exercise 2:_____	Weight:_____	Reps/Time:_____	Set 2:_____	Set 3:_____
Exercise 3:_____	Weight:_____	Reps/Time:_____	Set 2:_____	Set 3:_____
Exercise 4:_____	Weight:_____	Reps/Time:_____	Set 2:_____	Set 3:_____
Exercise 5:_____	Weight:_____	Reps/Time:_____	Set 2:_____	Set 3:_____
Exercise 6:_____	Weight:_____	Reps/Time:_____	Set 2:_____	Set 3:_____

Comments:_____
_____
_____
_____
_____

Workout:_____

Location:_____ Distance:_____ Duration:_____

Comments:_____
_____
_____
_____

SUMMARY

Tomorrow:_____

This Week:_____ This Month:_____

Wins:_____

Challenges:_____

Comments:_____
_____
_____
_____
_____

One Word   Success Score (1-10)

DAY 62
WEEK 9

DATE
/ /

1 - 10 SCORE

Energy:	"Big M":	Health:	Mood:	Stress:

DIET   Success Score:_____

Meals:_____
_____
_____
_____
_____

DATA

Weight:	Fat %:	x1: _____	x2: _____

MACRONUTRIENT CALCULATIONS

Carbs:	Protein:	Fat:	Calories:

_____
_____
_____
_____

Snacks:_____
_____

Comments:_____
_____
_____
_____

PRIMAL LIFESTYLE   Success Score:_____

Sleep (1-10):_____   Comments:_____
Sun (1-10):_____   Comments:_____
Play (1-10):_____   Comments:_____
Brain (1-10):_____   Comments:_____
Move (1-10):_____   Comments:_____

PERSONAL

Comments:_____
_____
_____
_____

EXERCISE   Success Score:_____   Effort Score:_____

Workout:_____

Location:_____ Duration:_____

Exercise 1:_____Weight:_____Reps/Time:_____Set 2:_____Set 3:_____

Exercise 2:_____Weight:_____Reps/Time:_____Set 2:_____Set 3:_____

Exercise 3:_____Weight:_____Reps/Time:_____Set 2:_____Set 3:_____

Exercise 4:_____Weight:_____Reps/Time:_____Set 2:_____Set 3:_____

Exercise 5:_____Weight:_____Reps/Time:_____Set 2:_____Set 3:_____

Exercise 6:_____Weight:_____Reps/Time:_____Set 2:_____Set 3:_____

Comments:_____

_____

_____

_____

_____

Workout:_____

Location:_____ Distance:_____ Duration:_____

Comments:_____

_____

_____

_____

SUMMARY

Tomorrow:_____

This Week:_____ This Month:_____

Wins:_____

Challenges:_____

Comments:_____

_____

_____

_____

_____

_____

One Word   Success Score (1-10)

DAY 63
WEEK 9

DATE ___/___/___

1 - 10 SCORE

Energy:	"Big M":	Health:	Mood:	Stress:

DIET

Success Score:_____

Meals:_____

_____

_____

_____

_____

DATA

Weight:	Fat %:	x1: _____	x2: _____

MACRONUTRIENT CALCULATIONS

Carbs:	Protein:	Fat:	Calories:

_____

_____

_____

_____

Snacks:_____

_____

Comments:_____

_____

_____

_____

PRIMAL LIFESTYLE

Success Score:_____

Sleep (1-10):_____ Comments:_____
Sun (1-10):_____ Comments:_____
Play (1-10):_____ Comments:_____
Brain (1-10):_____ Comments:_____
Move (1-10):_____ Comments:_____

PERSONAL

Comments:_____

_____

_____

_____

EXERCISE   Success Score:_____   Effort Score:_____

Workout:_____

Location:_____   Duration:_____

Exercise 1:	Weight:	Reps/Time:	Set 2:	Set 3:
Exercise 2:	Weight:	Reps/Time:	Set 2:	Set 3:
Exercise 3:	Weight:	Reps/Time:	Set 2:	Set 3:
Exercise 4:	Weight:	Reps/Time:	Set 2:	Set 3:
Exercise 5:	Weight:	Reps/Time:	Set 2:	Set 3:
Exercise 6:	Weight:	Reps/Time:	Set 2:	Set 3:

Comments:_____

_____

_____

_____

_____

Workout:_____

Location:_____   Distance:_____   Duration:_____

Comments:_____

_____

_____

_____

SUMMARY

Tomorrow:_____

This Week:_____   This Month:_____

Wins:_____

Challenges:_____

Comments:_____

_____

_____

_____

_____

One Word	Success Score (1-10)

DAY 64
WEEK 10

1 - 10 SCORE

Energy:	"Big M":	Health:	Mood:	Stress:

DIET

Success Score:_____

Meals:_____

_____

_____

_____

DATA

Weight:	Fat %:	x1: _____	x2: _____

MACRONUTRIENT CALCULATIONS

Carbs:	Protein:	Fat:	Calories:

_____

_____

_____

_____

Snacks:_____

Comments:_____

_____

_____

_____

PRIMAL LIFESTYLE

Success Score:_____

Sleep (1-10):_____ Comments:_____

Sun (1-10):_____ Comments:_____

Play (1-10):_____ Comments:_____

Brain (1-10):_____ Comments:_____

Move (1-10):_____ Comments:_____

PERSONAL

Comments:_____

_____

_____

_____

EXERCISE

Success Score:_____ Effort Score:_____

Workout:_____

Location:_____ Duration:_____

Exercise 1:_____ Weight:_____ Reps/Time:_____ Set 2:_____ Set 3:_____

Exercise 2:_____ Weight:_____ Reps/Time:_____ Set 2:_____ Set 3:_____

Exercise 3:_____ Weight:_____ Reps/Time:_____ Set 2:_____ Set 3:_____

Exercise 4:_____ Weight:_____ Reps/Time:_____ Set 2:_____ Set 3:_____

Exercise 5:_____ Weight:_____ Reps/Time:_____ Set 2:_____ Set 3:_____

Exercise 6:_____ Weight:_____ Reps/Time:_____ Set 2:_____ Set 3:_____

Comments:_____

_____

_____

_____

Workout:_____

Location:_____ Distance:_____ Duration:_____

Comments:_____

_____

_____

_____

SUMMARY

Tomorrow:_____

This Week:_____ This Month:_____

Wins:_____

Challenges:_____

Comments:_____

_____

_____

_____

_____

One Word   Success Score (1-10)

DAY 65
WEEK 10

DATE ___ / ___ / ___

Energy:	"Big M":	Health:	Mood:	Stress:

DIET   Success Score:_____

Meals:_____

_____

_____

_____

_____

DATA

Weight:	Fat %:	x1: _____	x2: _____

MACRONUTRIENT CALCULATIONS

Carbs:	Protein:	Fat:	Calories:

_____

_____

_____

_____

Snacks:_____

Comments:_____

_____

_____

_____

PRIMAL LIFESTYLE   Success Score:_____

Sleep (1-10):_____ Comments:_____

Sun (1-10):_____ Comments:_____

Play (1-10):_____ Comments:_____

Brain (1-10):_____ Comments:_____

Move (1-10):_____ Comments:_____

PERSONAL

Comments:_____

_____

_____

_____

EXERCISE   Success Score:_____   Effort Score:_____

Workout:_____

Location:_____ Duration:_____

Exercise 1:_____ Weight:_____ Reps/Time:_____ Set 2:_____ Set 3:_____
Exercise 2:_____ Weight:_____ Reps/Time:_____ Set 2:_____ Set 3:_____
Exercise 3:_____ Weight:_____ Reps/Time:_____ Set 2:_____ Set 3:_____
Exercise 4:_____ Weight:_____ Reps/Time:_____ Set 2:_____ Set 3:_____
Exercise 5:_____ Weight:_____ Reps/Time:_____ Set 2:_____ Set 3:_____
Exercise 6:_____ Weight:_____ Reps/Time:_____ Set 2:_____ Set 3:_____

Comments:_____
_____
_____
_____
_____

Workout:_____

Location:_____ Distance:_____ Duration:_____

Comments:_____
_____
_____
_____

SUMMARY

Tomorrow:_____

This Week:_____ This Month:_____

Wins:_____

Challenges:_____

Comments:_____
_____
_____
_____
_____

One Word   Success Score (1-10)

DAY 66
WEEK 10

1 - 10 SCORE

Energy:	"Big M":	Health:	Mood:	Stress:

DIET   Success Score:_____

DATA

Weight:	Fat %:	x1: _____	x2: _____

Meals:_____

_____

MACRONUTRIENT CALCULATIONS

Carbs:	Protein:	Fat:	Calories:

_____

_____

_____

_____

_____

_____

_____

Snacks:_____

_____

Comments:_____

_____

_____

_____

PRIMAL LIFESTYLE   Success Score:_____

Sleep (1-10):_____ Comments:_____
Sun (1-10):_____ Comments:_____
Play (1-10):_____ Comments:_____
Brain (1-10):_____ Comments:_____
Move (1-10):_____ Comments:_____

PERSONAL

Comments:_____

_____

_____

_____

EXERCISE

Success Score:_____   Effort Score:_____

Workout:_____

Location:_____   Duration:_____

Exercise 1:_____ Weight:_____ Reps/Time:_____ Set 2:_____ Set 3:_____

Exercise 2:_____ Weight:_____ Reps/Time:_____ Set 2:_____ Set 3:_____

Exercise 3:_____ Weight:_____ Reps/Time:_____ Set 2:_____ Set 3:_____

Exercise 4:_____ Weight:_____ Reps/Time:_____ Set 2:_____ Set 3:_____

Exercise 5:_____ Weight:_____ Reps/Time:_____ Set 2:_____ Set 3:_____

Exercise 6:_____ Weight:_____ Reps/Time:_____ Set 2:_____ Set 3:_____

Comments:_____

_____

_____

_____

_____

Workout:_____

Location:_____ Distance:_____ Duration:_____

Comments:_____

_____

_____

_____

_____

SUMMARY

Tomorrow:_____

This Week:_____   This Month:_____

Wins:_____

Challenges:_____

Comments:_____

_____

_____

_____

_____

One Word   Success Score (1-10)

DAY 67
WEEK 10

DATE ___/___/___

DIET   Success Score:_____

Meals:_____

_____

_____

_____

DATA

Weight:	Fat %:	x1: _____	x2: _____

MACRONUTRIENT CALCULATIONS

Carbs:	Protein:	Fat:	Calories:

_____

_____

_____

_____

Snacks:_____

_____

Comments:_____

_____

_____

_____

PRIMAL LIFESTYLE   Success Score:_____

Sleep (1-10):_____   Comments:_____

Sun (1-10):_____   Comments:_____

Play (1-10):_____   Comments:_____

Brain (1-10):_____   Comments:_____

Move (1-10):_____   Comments:_____

PERSONAL

Comments:_____

_____

_____

_____

EXERCISE   Success Score:_____   Effort Score:_____

Workout:_____

Location:_____ Duration:_____

Exercise 1:_____ Weight:_____ Reps/Time:_____ Set 2:_____ Set 3:_____

Exercise 2:_____ Weight:_____ Reps/Time:_____ Set 2:_____ Set 3:_____

Exercise 3:_____ Weight:_____ Reps/Time:_____ Set 2:_____ Set 3:_____

Exercise 4:_____ Weight:_____ Reps/Time:_____ Set 2:_____ Set 3:_____

Exercise 5:_____ Weight:_____ Reps/Time:_____ Set 2:_____ Set 3:_____

Exercise 6:_____ Weight:_____ Reps/Time:_____ Set 2:_____ Set 3:_____

Comments:_____

_____

_____

_____

_____

Workout:_____

Location:_____ Distance:_____ Duration:_____

Comments:_____

_____

_____

_____

SUMMARY

Tomorrow:_____

This Week:_____ This Month:_____

Wins:_____

Challenges:_____

Comments:_____

_____

_____

_____

_____

One Word   Success Score (1-10)

DAY 68
WEEK 10

DATE / /

1 - 10 SCORE

Energy:	"Big M":	Health:	Mood:	Stress:

DIET

Success Score:_____

Meals:_____

_____

_____

_____

_____

DATA

Weight:	Fat %:	x1: _____	x2: _____

MACRONUTRIENT CALCULATIONS

Carbs:	Protein:	Fat:	Calories:

_____

_____

_____

_____

_____

Snacks:_____

_____

Comments:_____

_____

_____

_____

PRIMAL LIFESTYLE

Success Score:_____

Sleep (1-10):_____ Comments:_____

Sun (1-10):_____ Comments:_____

Play (1-10):_____ Comments:_____

Brain (1-10):_____ Comments:_____

Move (1-10):_____ Comments:_____

PERSONAL

Comments:_____

_____

_____

_____

EXERCISE   Success Score:_____   Effort Score:_____

Workout:_____

Location:_____ Duration:_____

Exercise 1:_____ Weight:_____ Reps/Time:_____ Set 2:_____ Set 3:_____

Exercise 2:_____ Weight:_____ Reps/Time:_____ Set 2:_____ Set 3:_____

Exercise 3:_____ Weight:_____ Reps/Time:_____ Set 2:_____ Set 3:_____

Exercise 4:_____ Weight:_____ Reps/Time:_____ Set 2:_____ Set 3:_____

Exercise 5:_____ Weight:_____ Reps/Time:_____ Set 2:_____ Set 3:_____

Exercise 6:_____ Weight:_____ Reps/Time:_____ Set 2:_____ Set 3:_____

Comments:_____

_____

_____

_____

_____

Workout:_____

Location:_____ Distance:_____ Duration:_____

Comments:_____

_____

_____

_____

SUMMARY

Tomorrow:_____

This Week:_____ This Month:_____

Wins:_____

Challenges:_____

Comments:_____

_____

_____

_____

_____

_____

One Word   Success Score (1-10)

DAY 69
WEEK 10

DATE
/ /

1 - 10 SCORE

Energy:	"Big M":	Health:	Mood:	Stress:

DIET   Success Score:_____

Meals:_____
_____
_____
_____
_____

DATA

Weight:	Fat %:	x1: _____	x2: _____

MACRONUTRIENT CALCULATIONS

Carbs:	Protein:	Fat:	Calories:

_____
_____
_____
_____

Snacks:_____
_____

Comments:_____
_____
_____
_____

PRIMAL LIFESTYLE   Success Score:_____

Sleep (1-10):_____ Comments:_____
Sun (1-10):_____ Comments:_____
Play (1-10):_____ Comments:_____
Brain (1-10):_____ Comments:_____
Move (1-10):_____ Comments:_____

PERSONAL

Comments:_____
_____
_____
_____

EXERCISE   Success Score:_____   Effort Score:_____

Workout:_____

Location:_____   Duration:_____

Exercise 1:_____Weight:_____Reps/Time:_____Set 2:_____Set 3:_____

Exercise 2:_____Weight:_____Reps/Time:_____Set 2:_____Set 3:_____

Exercise 3:_____Weight:_____Reps/Time:_____Set 2:_____Set 3:_____

Exercise 4:_____Weight:_____Reps/Time:_____Set 2:_____Set 3:_____

Exercise 5:_____Weight:_____Reps/Time:_____Set 2:_____Set 3:_____

Exercise 6:_____Weight:_____Reps/Time:_____Set 2:_____Set 3:_____

Comments:_____
_____
_____
_____
_____

Workout:_____

Location:_____   Distance:_____   Duration:_____

Comments:_____
_____
_____
_____

SUMMARY

Tomorrow:_____

This Week:_____   This Month:_____

Wins:_____

Challenges:_____

Comments:_____
_____
_____
_____

One Word   Success Score (1-10)

DAY 70
WEEK 10

DATE / /

1 - 10 SCORE

Energy:	"Big M":	Health:	Mood:	Stress:

DIET

Success Score:_____

Meals:_____

_____

_____

_____

DATA

Weight:	Fat %:	x1: _____	x2: _____

MACRONUTRIENT CALCULATIONS

Carbs:	Protein:	Fat:	Calories:

_____

_____

_____

_____

Snacks:_____

_____

Comments:_____

_____

_____

_____

PRIMAL LIFESTYLE

Success Score:_____

Sleep (1-10):_____ Comments:_____

Sun (1-10):_____ Comments:_____

Play (1-10):_____ Comments:_____

Brain (1-10):_____ Comments:_____

Move (1-10):_____ Comments:_____

PERSONAL

Comments:_____

_____

_____

_____

EXERCISE

Success Score:_____   Effort Score:_____

Workout:_____

Location:_____ Duration:_____

Exercise 1:_____Weight:_____Reps/Time:_____Set 2:_____Set 3:_____

Exercise 2:_____Weight:_____Reps/Time:_____Set 2:_____Set 3:_____

Exercise 3:_____Weight:_____Reps/Time:_____Set 2:_____Set 3:_____

Exercise 4:_____Weight:_____Reps/Time:_____Set 2:_____Set 3:_____

Exercise 5:_____Weight:_____Reps/Time:_____Set 2:_____Set 3:_____

Exercise 6:_____Weight:_____Reps/Time:_____Set 2:_____Set 3:_____

Comments:_____

_____

_____

_____

_____

Workout:_____

Location:_____ Distance:_____ Duration:_____

Comments:_____

_____

_____

_____

_____

SUMMARY

Tomorrow:_____

This Week:_____ This Month:_____

Wins:_____

Challenges:_____

Comments:_____

_____

_____

_____

_____

_____

One Word   Success Score (1-10)

DAY 71
WEEK 11

DATE
/ /

1 - 10 SCORE

Energy:	"Big M":	Health:	Mood:	Stress:

DIET   Success Score:_____

Meals:_____

_____

_____

_____

_____

DATA

Weight:	Fat %:	x1: _____	x2: _____

MACRONUTRIENT CALCULATIONS

Carbs:	Protein:	Fat:	Calories:

_____

_____

_____

_____

Snacks:_____

_____

Comments:_____

_____

_____

_____

PRIMAL LIFESTYLE   Success Score:_____

Sleep (1-10):_____   Comments:_____
Sun (1-10):_____   Comments:_____
Play (1-10):_____   Comments:_____
Brain (1-10):_____   Comments:_____
Move (1-10):_____   Comments:_____

PERSONAL

Comments:_____

_____

_____

_____

EXERCISE   Success Score:_____   Effort Score:_____

Workout:_____

Location:_____   Duration:_____

Exercise 1:_____ Weight:_____ Reps/Time:_____ Set 2:_____ Set 3:_____

Exercise 2:_____ Weight:_____ Reps/Time:_____ Set 2:_____ Set 3:_____

Exercise 3:_____ Weight:_____ Reps/Time:_____ Set 2:_____ Set 3:_____

Exercise 4:_____ Weight:_____ Reps/Time:_____ Set 2:_____ Set 3:_____

Exercise 5:_____ Weight:_____ Reps/Time:_____ Set 2:_____ Set 3:_____

Exercise 6:_____ Weight:_____ Reps/Time:_____ Set 2:_____ Set 3:_____

Comments:_____

_____

_____

_____

_____

Workout:_____

Location:_____ Distance:_____ Duration:_____

Comments:_____

_____

_____

_____

_____

SUMMARY

Tomorrow:_____

This Week:_____   This Month:_____

Wins:_____

Challenges:_____

Comments:_____

_____

_____

_____

_____

_____

One Word   Success Score (1-10)

DAY 72
WEEK 11

1 - 10 SCORE

Energy:	"Big M":	Health:	Mood:	Stress:

DIET   Success Score:_____

Meals:_____

_____

DATA

Weight:	Fat %:	x1: _____	x2: _____

_____

MACRONUTRIENT CALCULATIONS

Carbs:	Protein:	Fat:	Calories:

_____

_____

_____

_____

_____

Snacks:_____

Comments:_____

_____

_____

_____

PRIMAL LIFESTYLE   Success Score:_____

Sleep (1-10):_____ Comments:_____

Sun (1-10):_____ Comments:_____

Play (1-10):_____ Comments:_____

Brain (1-10):_____ Comments:_____

Move (1-10):_____ Comments:_____

PERSONAL

Comments:_____

_____

_____

_____

EXERCISE   Success Score:_____   Effort Score:_____

Workout:_____

Location:_____ Duration:_____

Exercise 1:_____Weight:_____ Reps/Time:_____ Set 2:_____ Set 3:_____

Exercise 2:_____Weight:_____ Reps/Time:_____ Set 2:_____ Set 3:_____

Exercise 3:_____Weight:_____ Reps/Time:_____ Set 2:_____ Set 3:_____

Exercise 4:_____Weight:_____ Reps/Time:_____ Set 2:_____ Set 3:_____

Exercise 5:_____Weight:_____ Reps/Time:_____ Set 2:_____ Set 3:_____

Exercise 6:_____Weight:_____ Reps/Time:_____ Set 2:_____ Set 3:_____

Comments:_____

_____

_____

_____

_____

Workout:_____

Location:_____ Distance:_____ Duration:_____

Comments:_____

_____

_____

_____

_____

SUMMARY

Tomorrow:_____

This Week:_____ This Month:_____

Wins:_____

Challenges:_____

Comments:_____

_____

_____

_____

One Word   Success Score (1-10)

DAY 73
WEEK 11

DATE
/ /

1 - 10 SCORE

Energy:	"Big M":	Health:	Mood:	Stress:

DIET

Success Score:_____

Meals:_____

_____

_____

_____

_____

DATA

Weight:	Fat %:	x1: _____	x2: _____

MACRONUTRIENT CALCULATIONS

Carbs:	Protein:	Fat:	Calories:

_____

_____

_____

_____

Snacks:_____

_____

Comments:_____

_____

_____

_____

PRIMAL LIFESTYLE

Success Score:_____

Sleep (1-10):_____ Comments:_____

Sun (1-10):_____ Comments:_____

Play (1-10):_____ Comments:_____

Brain (1-10):_____ Comments:_____

Move (1-10):_____ Comments:_____

PERSONAL

Comments:_____

_____

_____

_____

Success Score:_____   Effort Score:_____

Workout:_____

Location:_____ Duration:_____

Exercise 1:_____ Weight:_____ Reps/Time:_____ Set 2:_____ Set 3:_____

Exercise 2:_____ Weight:_____ Reps/Time:_____ Set 2:_____ Set 3:_____

Exercise 3:_____ Weight:_____ Reps/Time:_____ Set 2:_____ Set 3:_____

Exercise 4:_____ Weight:_____ Reps/Time:_____ Set 2:_____ Set 3:_____

Exercise 5:_____ Weight:_____ Reps/Time:_____ Set 2:_____ Set 3:_____

Exercise 6:_____ Weight:_____ Reps/Time:_____ Set 2:_____ Set 3:_____

Comments:_____

_____

_____

_____

_____

Workout:_____

Location:_____ Distance:_____ Duration:_____

Comments:_____

_____

_____

_____

_____

SUMMARY

Tomorrow:_____

This Week:_____ This Month:_____ _____

Wins:_____

Challenges:_____

Comments:_____

_____

_____

_____

_____

One Word   Success Score (1-10)

DAY 74
WEEK 11

DATE / /

1 - 10 SCORE

Energy:	"Big M":	Health:	Mood:	Stress:

DIET   Success Score:_____

DATA

Weight:	Fat %:	x1: _____	x2: _____

Meals:_____

_____

_____

_____

MACRONUTRIENT CALCULATIONS

Carbs:	Protein:	Fat:	Calories:

_____

_____

_____

_____

Snacks:_____

_____

Comments:_____

_____

_____

_____

PRIMAL LIFESTYLE   Success Score:_____

Sleep (1-10):_____   Comments:_____

Sun (1-10):_____   Comments:_____

Play (1-10):_____   Comments:_____

Brain (1-10):_____   Comments:_____

Move (1-10):_____   Comments:_____

PERSONAL

Comments:_____

_____

_____

_____

EXERCISE   Success Score:_____   Effort Score:_____

Workout:_____

Location:_____ Duration:_____

Exercise 1:_____ Weight:_____ Reps/Time:_____ Set 2:_____ Set 3:_____

Exercise 2:_____ Weight:_____ Reps/Time:_____ Set 2:_____ Set 3:_____

Exercise 3:_____ Weight:_____ Reps/Time:_____ Set 2:_____ Set 3:_____

Exercise 4:_____ Weight:_____ Reps/Time:_____ Set 2:_____ Set 3:_____

Exercise 5:_____ Weight:_____ Reps/Time:_____ Set 2:_____ Set 3:_____

Exercise 6:_____ Weight:_____ Reps/Time:_____ Set 2:_____ Set 3:_____

Comments:_____

_____

_____

_____

Workout:_____

Location:_____ Distance:_____ Duration:_____

Comments:_____

_____

_____

_____

SUMMARY

Tomorrow:_____

This Week:_____ This Month:_____

Wins:_____

Challenges:_____

Comments:_____

_____

_____

One Word   Success Score (1-10)

DAY 75
WEEK 11

DATE / /

1 - 10 SCORE

Energy:	"Big M":	Health:	Mood:	Stress:

DIET

Success Score:_____

Meals:_____

_____

_____

_____

_____

DATA

Weight:	Fat %:	x1: _____	x2: _____

MACRONUTRIENT CALCULATIONS

Carbs:	Protein:	Fat:	Calories:

_____

_____

_____

_____

Snacks:_____

_____

Comments:_____

_____

_____

PRIMAL LIFESTYLE

Success Score:_____

Sleep (1-10):_____ Comments:_____

Sun (1-10):_____ Comments:_____

Play (1-10):_____ Comments:_____

Brain (1-10):_____ Comments:_____

Move (1-10):_____ Comments:_____

PERSONAL

Comments:_____

_____

_____

_____

EXERCISE   Success Score:_____ Effort Score:_____

Workout:_____

Location:_____ Duration:_____

Exercise 1:_____ Weight:_____ Reps/Time:_____ Set 2:_____ Set 3:_____

Exercise 2:_____ Weight:_____ Reps/Time:_____ Set 2:_____ Set 3:_____

Exercise 3:_____ Weight:_____ Reps/Time:_____ Set 2:_____ Set 3:_____

Exercise 4:_____ Weight:_____ Reps/Time:_____ Set 2:_____ Set 3:_____

Exercise 5:_____ Weight:_____ Reps/Time:_____ Set 2:_____ Set 3:_____

Exercise 6:_____ Weight:_____ Reps/Time:_____ Set 2:_____ Set 3:_____

Comments:_____

_____

_____

_____

_____

Workout:_____

Location:_____ Distance:_____ Duration:_____

Comments:_____

_____

_____

_____

SUMMARY

Tomorrow:_____

This Week:_____ This Month:_____

Wins:_____

Challenges:_____

Comments:_____

_____

_____

_____

_____

One Word   Success Score (1-10)

DAY 76
WEEK 11

DATE
/ /

1 - 10 SCORE

Energy:	"Big M":	Health:	Mood:	Stress:

DIET   Success Score:_____

DATA

Weight:	Fat %:	x1: _____	x2: _____

Meals:_____

_____

_____

MACRONUTRIENT CALCULATIONS

Carbs:	Protein:	Fat:	Calories:

_____

_____

_____

_____

_____

Snacks:_____

_____

Comments:_____

_____

_____

_____

PRIMAL LIFESTYLE   Success Score:_____

Sleep (1-10):_____   Comments:_____
Sun (1-10):_____   Comments:_____
Play (1-10):_____   Comments:_____
Brain (1-10):_____   Comments:_____
Move (1-10):_____   Comments:_____

PERSONAL

Comments:_____

_____

_____

_____

EXERCISE   Success Score:_____   Effort Score:_____

Workout:_____

Location:_____ Duration:_____

Exercise 1:	Weight:	Reps/Time:	Set 2:	Set 3:
Exercise 2:	Weight:	Reps/Time:	Set 2:	Set 3:
Exercise 3:	Weight:	Reps/Time:	Set 2:	Set 3:
Exercise 4:	Weight:	Reps/Time:	Set 2:	Set 3:
Exercise 5:	Weight:	Reps/Time:	Set 2:	Set 3:
Exercise 6:	Weight:	Reps/Time:	Set 2:	Set 3:

Comments:_____

_____

_____

_____

_____

Workout:_____

Location:_____ Distance:_____ Duration:_____

Comments:_____

_____

_____

_____

SUMMARY

Tomorrow:_____

This Week:_____ This Month:_____

Wins:_____

Challenges:_____

Comments:_____

_____

_____

_____   [   ]   [   ]

_____

_____   One Word   Success Score (1-10)

DAY 77
WEEK 11

DATE / /

1 - 10 SCORE

Energy:	"Big M":	Health:	Mood:	Stress:

DIET

Success Score:_____

Meals:_____

_____

_____

_____

_____

DATA

Weight:	Fat %:	x1: _____	x2: _____

MACRONUTRIENT CALCULATIONS

Carbs:	Protein:	Fat:	Calories:

_____

_____

_____

_____

Snacks:_____

_____

Comments:_____

_____

_____

_____

PRIMAL LIFESTYLE

Success Score:_____

Sleep (1-10):_____ Comments:_____

Sun (1-10):_____ Comments:_____

Play (1-10):_____ Comments:_____

Brain (1-10):_____ Comments:_____

Move (1-10):_____ Comments:_____

PERSONAL

Comments:_____

_____

_____

_____

EXERCISE

Success Score:_____ Effort Score:_____

Workout:_____

Location:_____ Duration:_____

Exercise 1:_____Weight:_____ Reps/Time:_____ Set 2:_____ Set 3:_____

Exercise 2:_____Weight:_____ Reps/Time:_____ Set 2:_____ Set 3:_____

Exercise 3:_____Weight:_____ Reps/Time:_____ Set 2:_____ Set 3:_____

Exercise 4:_____Weight:_____ Reps/Time:_____ Set 2:_____ Set 3:_____

Exercise 5:_____Weight:_____ Reps/Time:_____ Set 2:_____ Set 3:_____

Exercise 6:_____Weight:_____ Reps/Time:_____ Set 2:_____ Set 3:_____

Comments:_____

_____

_____

_____

_____

Workout:_____

Location:_____ Distance:_____ Duration:_____

Comments:_____

_____

_____

_____

SUMMARY

Tomorrow:_____

This Week:_____ This Month:_____

Wins:_____

Challenges:_____

Comments:_____

_____

_____

_____

_____

_____

One Word   Success Score (1-10)

DAY 78
WEEK 12

DATE __ / __ / __

1 - 10 SCORE

Energy:	"Big M":	Health:	Mood:	Stress:

DIET

Success Score:_____

Meals:_____

_____

_____

_____

_____

DATA

Weight:	Fat %:	x1: _____	x2: _____

MACRONUTRIENT CALCULATIONS

Carbs:	Protein:	Fat:	Calories:

_____

_____

_____

_____

Snacks:_____

_____

Comments:_____

_____

_____

_____

PRIMAL LIFESTYLE

Success Score:_____

Sleep (1-10):_____ Comments:_____

Sun (1-10):_____ Comments:_____

Play (1-10):_____ Comments:_____

Brain (1-10):_____ Comments:_____

Move (1-10):_____ Comments:_____

PERSONAL

Comments:_____

_____

_____

_____

EXERCISE   Success Score:_____   Effort Score:_____

Workout:_____

Location:_____   Duration:_____

Exercise 1:_____ Weight:_____ Reps/Time:_____ Set 2:_____ Set 3:_____

Exercise 2:_____ Weight:_____ Reps/Time:_____ Set 2:_____ Set 3:_____

Exercise 3:_____ Weight:_____ Reps/Time:_____ Set 2:_____ Set 3:_____

Exercise 4:_____ Weight:_____ Reps/Time:_____ Set 2:_____ Set 3:_____

Exercise 5:_____ Weight:_____ Reps/Time:_____ Set 2:_____ Set 3:_____

Exercise 6:_____ Weight:_____ Reps/Time:_____ Set 2:_____ Set 3:_____

Comments:_____

_____

_____

_____

_____

Workout:_____

Location:_____ Distance:_____ Duration:_____

Comments:_____

_____

_____

_____

SUMMARY

Tomorrow:_____

This Week:_____ This Month:_____

Wins:_____

Challenges:_____

Comments:_____

_____

_____

_____

_____

_____ | | | |

One Word   Success Score (1-10)

DAY 79
WEEK 12

DATE __/__/__

Energy:	"Big M":	Health:	Mood:	Stress:

DIET

Success Score:_____

Meals:_____
_____
_____
_____
_____

DATA

Weight:	Fat %:	x1: _____	x2: _____

MACRONUTRIENT CALCULATIONS

Carbs:	Protein:	Fat:	Calories:

_____
_____
_____
_____
_____

Snacks:_____
_____

Comments:_____
_____
_____
_____

PRIMAL LIFESTYLE

Success Score:_____

Sleep (1-10):_____ Comments:_____
Sun (1-10):_____ Comments:_____
Play (1-10):_____ Comments:_____
Brain (1-10):_____ Comments:_____
Move (1-10):_____ Comments:_____

PERSONAL

Comments:_____
_____
_____
_____

EXERCISE Success Score:_____ Effort Score:_____

Workout:_____

Location:_____ Duration:_____

Exercise 1:_____ Weight:_____ Reps/Time:_____ Set 2:_____ Set 3:_____

Exercise 2:_____ Weight:_____ Reps/Time:_____ Set 2:_____ Set 3:_____

Exercise 3:_____ Weight:_____ Reps/Time:_____ Set 2:_____ Set 3:_____

Exercise 4:_____ Weight:_____ Reps/Time:_____ Set 2:_____ Set 3:_____

Exercise 5:_____ Weight:_____ Reps/Time:_____ Set 2:_____ Set 3:_____

Exercise 6:_____ Weight:_____ Reps/Time:_____ Set 2:_____ Set 3:_____

Comments:_____

_____

_____

_____

_____

Workout:_____

Location:_____ Distance:_____ Duration:_____

Comments:_____

_____

_____

_____

_____

SUMMARY

Tomorrow:_____

This Week:_____ This Month:_____

Wins:_____

Challenges:_____

Comments:_____

_____

_____

_____

_____

_____

One Word   Success Score (1-10)

DAY 80
WEEK 12

DATE ___ / ___ / ___

1 - 10 SCORE

Energy:	"Big M":	Health:	Mood:	Stress:

DIET   Success Score:_____

Meals:_____

_____

_____

_____

_____

DATA

Weight:	Fat %:	x1: _____	x2: _____

MACRONUTRIENT CALCULATIONS

Carbs:	Protein:	Fat:	Calories:

_____

_____

_____

_____

Snacks:_____

_____

Comments:_____

_____

_____

_____

PRIMAL LIFESTYLE   Success Score:_____

Sleep (1-10):_____   Comments:_____

Sun (1-10):_____   Comments:_____

Play (1-10):_____   Comments:_____

Brain (1-10):_____   Comments:_____

Move (1-10):_____   Comments:_____

PERSONAL

Comments:_____

_____

_____

_____

EXERCISE   Success Score:_____   Effort Score:_____

Workout:_____

Location:_____ Duration:_____

Exercise 1:_____Weight:_____ Reps/Time:_____ Set 2:_____ Set 3:_____

Exercise 2:_____Weight:_____ Reps/Time:_____ Set 2:_____ Set 3:_____

Exercise 3:_____Weight:_____ Reps/Time:_____ Set 2:_____ Set 3:_____

Exercise 4:_____Weight:_____ Reps/Time:_____ Set 2:_____ Set 3:_____

Exercise 5:_____Weight:_____ Reps/Time:_____ Set 2:_____ Set 3:_____

Exercise 6:_____Weight:_____ Reps/Time:_____ Set 2:_____ Set 3:_____

Comments:_____

_____

_____

_____

_____

Workout:_____

Location:_____ Distance:_____ Duration:_____

Comments:_____

_____

_____

_____

_____

SUMMARY

Tomorrow:_____

This Week:_____ This Month:_____

Wins:_____

Challenges:_____

Comments:_____

_____

_____

_____

_____

One Word   Success Score (1-10)

DAY 81
WEEK 12

DATE

/ /

1 - 10 SCORE

Energy:	"Big M":	Health:	Mood:	Stress:

DIET

Success Score:_____

Meals:_____
_____
_____
_____
_____

DATA

Weight:	Fat %:	x1: _____	x2: _____

MACRONUTRIENT CALCULATIONS

Carbs:	Protein:	Fat:	Calories:

_____
_____
_____
_____
_____

Snacks:_____
_____

Comments:_____
_____
_____
_____

PRIMAL LIFESTYLE

Success Score:_____

Sleep (1-10):_____ Comments:_____
Sun (1-10):_____ Comments:_____
Play (1-10):_____ Comments:_____
Brain (1-10):_____ Comments:_____
Move (1-10):_____ Comments:_____

PERSONAL

Comments:_____
_____
_____
_____

EXERCISE

Success Score:_____ Effort Score:_____

Workout:_____

Location:_____ Duration:_____

Exercise 1:_____ Weight:_____ Reps/Time:_____ Set 2:_____ Set 3:_____

Exercise 2:_____ Weight:_____ Reps/Time:_____ Set 2:_____ Set 3:_____

Exercise 3:_____ Weight:_____ Reps/Time:_____ Set 2:_____ Set 3:_____

Exercise 4:_____ Weight:_____ Reps/Time:_____ Set 2:_____ Set 3:_____

Exercise 5:_____ Weight:_____ Reps/Time:_____ Set 2:_____ Set 3:_____

Exercise 6:_____ Weight:_____ Reps/Time:_____ Set 2:_____ Set 3:_____

Comments:_____

_____

_____

_____

_____

Workout:_____

Location:_____ Distance:_____ Duration:_____

Comments:_____

_____

_____

_____

SUMMARY

Tomorrow:_____

This Week:_____ This Month:_____

Wins:_____

Challenges:_____

Comments:_____

_____

_____

_____

_____

_____

One Word   Success Score (1-10)

DAY 82
WEEK 12

DATE ___/___/___

1 - 10 SCORE

Energy:	"Big M":	Health:	Mood:	Stress:

DIET   Success Score:_____

Meals:_____

_____

_____

_____

DATA

Weight:	Fat %:	x1: _____	x2: _____

MACRONUTRIENT CALCULATIONS

Carbs:	Protein:	Fat:	Calories:

_____

_____

_____

_____

Snacks:_____

_____

Comments:_____

_____

_____

_____

PRIMAL LIFESTYLE   Success Score:_____

Sleep (1-10):_____   Comments:_____

Sun (1-10):_____   Comments:_____

Play (1-10):_____   Comments:_____

Brain (1-10):_____   Comments:_____

Move (1-10):_____   Comments:_____

PERSONAL

Comments:_____

_____

_____

_____

EXERCISE   Success Score:_____   Effort Score:_____

Workout:_____

Location:_____ Duration:_____

Exercise 1:	Weight:	Reps/Time:	Set 2:	Set 3:
Exercise 2:	Weight:	Reps/Time:	Set 2:	Set 3:
Exercise 3:	Weight:	Reps/Time:	Set 2:	Set 3:
Exercise 4:	Weight:	Reps/Time:	Set 2:	Set 3:
Exercise 5:	Weight:	Reps/Time:	Set 2:	Set 3:
Exercise 6:	Weight:	Reps/Time:	Set 2:	Set 3:

Comments:_____

_____

_____

_____

_____

_____

Workout:_____

Location:_____ Distance:_____ Duration:_____

Comments:_____

_____

_____

_____

_____

SUMMARY

Tomorrow:_____

This Week:_____ This Month:_____

Wins:_____

Challenges:_____

Comments:_____

_____

_____

_____

_____   One Word   Success Score (1-10)

_____

DAY 83
WEEK 12

DATE ___/___/___

1 - 10 SCORE

Energy:	"Big M":	Health:	Mood:	Stress:

DIET   Success Score:_____

DATA

Weight:	Fat %:	x1: _____	x2: _____

Meals:_____

_____

MACRONUTRIENT CALCULATIONS

Carbs:	Protein:	Fat:	Calories:

_____

_____

_____

_____

_____

_____

_____

Snacks:_____

_____

Comments:_____

_____

_____

_____

PRIMAL LIFESTYLE   Success Score:_____

Sleep (1-10):_____   Comments:_____

Sun (1-10):_____   Comments:_____

Play (1-10):_____   Comments:_____

Brain (1-10):_____   Comments:_____

Move (1-10):_____   Comments:_____

PERSONAL

Comments:_____

_____

_____

_____

EXERCISE   Success Score:_____   Effort Score:_____

Workout:_____

Location:_____ Duration:_____

Exercise 1:_____ Weight:_____ Reps/Time:_____ Set 2:_____ Set 3:_____

Exercise 2:_____ Weight:_____ Reps/Time:_____ Set 2:_____ Set 3:_____

Exercise 3:_____ Weight:_____ Reps/Time:_____ Set 2:_____ Set 3:_____

Exercise 4:_____ Weight:_____ Reps/Time:_____ Set 2:_____ Set 3:_____

Exercise 5:_____ Weight:_____ Reps/Time:_____ Set 2:_____ Set 3:_____

Exercise 6:_____ Weight:_____ Reps/Time:_____ Set 2:_____ Set 3:_____

Comments:_____

_____

_____

_____

_____

Workout:_____

Location:_____ Distance:_____ Duration:_____

Comments:_____

_____

_____

_____

_____

SUMMARY

Tomorrow:_____

This Week:_____ This Month:_____

Wins:_____

Challenges:_____

Comments:_____

_____

_____

_____

_____

One Word   Success Score (1-10)

DAY 84
WEEK 12

DATE / /

Energy:	"Big M":	Health:	Mood:	Stress:

DIET

Success Score:_____

Meals:_____

_____

_____

_____

DATA

Weight:	Fat %:	x1: _____	x2: _____

MACRONUTRIENT CALCULATIONS

Carbs:	Protein:	Fat:	Calories:

_____

_____

_____

_____

Snacks:_____

_____

Comments:_____

_____

_____

PRIMAL LIFESTYLE

Success Score:_____

Sleep (1-10):_____ Comments:_____

Sun (1-10):_____ Comments:_____

Play (1-10):_____ Comments:_____

Brain (1-10):_____ Comments:_____

Move (1-10):_____ Comments:_____

PERSONAL

Comments:_____

_____

_____

_____

EXERCISE   Success Score:_____   Effort Score:_____

Workout:_____

Location:_____ Duration:_____

Exercise 1:_____ Weight:_____ Reps/Time:_____ Set 2:_____ Set 3:_____

Exercise 2:_____ Weight:_____ Reps/Time:_____ Set 2:_____ Set 3:_____

Exercise 3:_____ Weight:_____ Reps/Time:_____ Set 2:_____ Set 3:_____

Exercise 4:_____ Weight:_____ Reps/Time:_____ Set 2:_____ Set 3:_____

Exercise 5:_____ Weight:_____ Reps/Time:_____ Set 2:_____ Set 3:_____

Exercise 6:_____ Weight:_____ Reps/Time:_____ Set 2:_____ Set 3:_____

Comments:_____

_____

_____

_____

_____

Workout:_____

Location:_____ Distance:_____ Duration:_____

Comments:_____

_____

_____

_____

_____

SUMMARY

Tomorrow:_____

This Week:_____ This Month:_____

Wins:_____

Challenges:_____

Comments:_____

_____

_____

_____

_____

One Word   Success Score (1-10)

DAY 85
WEEK 13

DATE
/ /

1 - 10 SCORE

Energy:	"Big M":	Health:	Mood:	Stress:

DIET   Success Score:_____

Meals:_____

_____

_____

_____

DATA

Weight:	Fat %:	x1: _____	x2: _____

MACRONUTRIENT CALCULATIONS

Carbs:	Protein:	Fat:	Calories:

_____

_____

_____

_____

Snacks:_____

_____

Comments:_____

_____

_____

_____

PRIMAL LIFESTYLE   Success Score:_____

Sleep (1-10):_____ Comments:_____

Sun (1-10):_____ Comments:_____

Play (1-10):_____ Comments:_____

Brain (1-10):_____ Comments:_____

Move (1-10):_____ Comments:_____

PERSONAL

Comments:_____

_____

_____

_____

EXERCISE

Success Score:_____ Effort Score:_____

Workout:_____

Location:_____ Duration:_____

Exercise 1:_____ Weight:_____ Reps/Time:_____ Set 2:_____ Set 3:_____

Exercise 2:_____ Weight:_____ Reps/Time:_____ Set 2:_____ Set 3:_____

Exercise 3:_____ Weight:_____ Reps/Time:_____ Set 2:_____ Set 3:_____

Exercise 4:_____ Weight:_____ Reps/Time:_____ Set 2:_____ Set 3:_____

Exercise 5:_____ Weight:_____ Reps/Time:_____ Set 2:_____ Set 3:_____

Exercise 6:_____ Weight:_____ Reps/Time:_____ Set 2:_____ Set 3:_____

Comments:_____
_____
_____
_____

Workout:_____

Location:_____ Distance:_____ Duration:_____

Comments:_____
_____
_____
_____

SUMMARY

Tomorrow:_____

This Week:_____ This Month:_____

Wins:_____

Challenges:_____

Comments:_____
_____
_____
_____

One Word   Success Score (1-10)

DAY 86
WEEK 13

DATE ___ / ___ / ___

DIET   Success Score:_____

Meals:_____

_____

_____

_____

DATA

Weight:	Fat %:	x1: _____	x2: _____

MACRONUTRIENT CALCULATIONS

Carbs:	Protein:	Fat:	Calories:

_____

_____

_____

_____

Snacks:_____

Comments:_____

_____

_____

_____

PRIMAL LIFESTYLE   Success Score:_____

Sleep (1-10):_____   Comments:_____

Sun (1-10):_____   Comments:_____

Play (1-10):_____   Comments:_____

Brain (1-10):_____   Comments:_____

Move (1-10):_____   Comments:_____

PERSONAL

Comments:_____

_____

_____

_____

EXERCISE   Success Score:_____   Effort Score:_____

Workout:_____

Location:_____   Duration:_____

Exercise 1:_____ Weight:_____ Reps/Time:_____ Set 2:_____ Set 3:_____

Exercise 2:_____ Weight:_____ Reps/Time:_____ Set 2:_____ Set 3:_____

Exercise 3:_____ Weight:_____ Reps/Time:_____ Set 2:_____ Set 3:_____

Exercise 4:_____ Weight:_____ Reps/Time:_____ Set 2:_____ Set 3:_____

Exercise 5:_____ Weight:_____ Reps/Time:_____ Set 2:_____ Set 3:_____

Exercise 6:_____ Weight:_____ Reps/Time:_____ Set 2:_____ Set 3:_____

Comments:_____

_____

_____

_____

_____

Workout:_____

Location:_____ Distance:_____ Duration:_____

Comments:_____

_____

_____

_____

SUMMARY

Tomorrow:_____

This Week:_____   This Month:_____

Wins:_____

Challenges:_____

Comments:_____

_____

_____

_____

_____

_____

One Word   Success Score (1-10)

DAY 87
WEEK 13

DATE / /

Energy:	"Big M":	Health:	Mood:	Stress:

DIET   Success Score:_____

Meals:_____

_____

_____

_____

DATA

Weight:	Fat %:	x1: _____	x2: _____

MACRONUTRIENT CALCULATIONS

Carbs:	Protein:	Fat:	Calories:

_____

_____

_____

_____

Snacks:_____

_____

Comments:_____

_____

_____

_____

PRIMAL LIFESTYLE   Success Score:_____

Sleep (1-10):_____   Comments:_____

Sun (1-10):_____   Comments:_____

Play (1-10):_____   Comments:_____

Brain (1-10):_____   Comments:_____

Move (1-10):_____   Comments:_____

PERSONAL

Comments:_____

_____

_____

_____

EXERCISE   Success Score:_____   Effort Score:_____

Workout:_____

Location:_____ Duration:_____

Exercise 1:_____ Weight:_____ Reps/Time:_____ Set 2:_____ Set 3:_____

Exercise 2:_____ Weight:_____ Reps/Time:_____ Set 2:_____ Set 3:_____

Exercise 3:_____ Weight:_____ Reps/Time:_____ Set 2:_____ Set 3:_____

Exercise 4:_____ Weight:_____ Reps/Time:_____ Set 2:_____ Set 3:_____

Exercise 5:_____ Weight:_____ Reps/Time:_____ Set 2:_____ Set 3:_____

Exercise 6:_____ Weight:_____ Reps/Time:_____ Set 2:_____ Set 3:_____

Comments:_____

_____

_____

_____

Workout:_____

Location:_____ Distance:_____ Duration:_____

Comments:_____

_____

_____

_____

SUMMARY

Tomorrow:_____

This Week:_____ This Month:_____

Wins:_____

Challenges:_____

Comments:_____

_____

_____

_____

_____

_____

One Word   Success Score (1-10)

DAY 88
WEEK 13

DATE ___ / ___ / ___

1 - 10 SCORE

Energy:	"Big M":	Health:	Mood:	Stress:

DIET   Success Score:_____

Meals:_____

_____

_____

_____

DATA

Weight:	Fat %:	x1: _____	x2: _____

MACRONUTRIENT CALCULATIONS

Carbs:	Protein:	Fat:	Calories:

_____

_____

_____

_____

Snacks:_____

Comments:_____

_____

_____

_____

PRIMAL LIFESTYLE   Success Score:_____

Sleep (1-10):_____   Comments:_____

Sun (1-10):_____   Comments:_____

Play (1-10):_____   Comments:_____

Brain (1-10):_____   Comments:_____

Move (1-10):_____   Comments:_____

PERSONAL

Comments:_____

_____

_____

_____

EXERCISE

Success Score:_____ Effort Score:_____

Workout:_____

Location:_____ Duration:_____

Exercise 1:_____ Weight:_____ Reps/Time:_____ Set 2:_____ Set 3:_____

Exercise 2:_____ Weight:_____ Reps/Time:_____ Set 2:_____ Set 3:_____

Exercise 3:_____ Weight:_____ Reps/Time:_____ Set 2:_____ Set 3:_____

Exercise 4:_____ Weight:_____ Reps/Time:_____ Set 2:_____ Set 3:_____

Exercise 5:_____ Weight:_____ Reps/Time:_____ Set 2:_____ Set 3:_____

Exercise 6:_____ Weight:_____ Reps/Time:_____ Set 2:_____ Set 3:_____

Comments:_____

_____

_____

_____

_____

Workout:_____

Location:_____ Distance:_____ Duration:_____

Comments:_____

_____

_____

_____

SUMMARY

Tomorrow:_____

This Week:_____ This Month:_____

Wins:_____

Challenges:_____

Comments:_____

_____

_____

_____   One Word   Success Score (1-10)

_____

_____

DAY 89
WEEK 13

DATE / /

1 - 10 SCORE

Energy:	"Big M":	Health:	Mood:	Stress:

DIET

Success Score:_____

Meals:_____
_____
_____
_____
_____

DATA

Weight:	Fat %:	x1: _____	x2: _____

MACRONUTRIENT CALCULATIONS

Carbs:	Protein:	Fat:	Calories:

_____
_____
_____
_____
_____

Snacks:_____
_____

Comments:_____
_____
_____
_____

PRIMAL LIFESTYLE   Success Score:_____

Sleep (1-10):_____   Comments:_____
Sun (1-10):_____   Comments:_____
Play (1-10):_____   Comments:_____
Brain (1-10):_____   Comments:_____
Move (1-10):_____   Comments:_____

PERSONAL

Comments:_____
_____
_____
_____

EXERCISE   Success Score:_____   Effort Score:_____

Workout:_____

Location:_____ Duration:_____

Exercise 1:_____ Weight:_____ Reps/Time:_____ Set 2:_____ Set 3:_____

Exercise 2:_____ Weight:_____ Reps/Time:_____ Set 2:_____ Set 3:_____

Exercise 3:_____ Weight:_____ Reps/Time:_____ Set 2:_____ Set 3:_____

Exercise 4:_____ Weight:_____ Reps/Time:_____ Set 2:_____ Set 3:_____

Exercise 5:_____ Weight:_____ Reps/Time:_____ Set 2:_____ Set 3:_____

Exercise 6:_____ Weight:_____ Reps/Time:_____ Set 2:_____ Set 3:_____

Comments:_____

_____

_____

_____

_____

Workout:_____

Location:_____ Distance:_____ Duration:_____

Comments:_____

_____

_____

_____

SUMMARY

Tomorrow:_____

This Week:_____ This Month:_____

Wins:_____

Challenges:_____

Comments:_____

_____

_____

_____

_____

_____

One Word   Success Score (1-10)

DAY 90

WEEK 13

DATE / /

1 - 10 SCORE

Energy:	"Big M":	Health:	Mood:	Stress:

DIET   Success Score:_____

Meals:_____

_____

_____

_____

DATA

Weight:	Fat %:	x1: _____	x2: _____

MACRONUTRIENT CALCULATIONS

Carbs:	Protein:	Fat:	Calories:

_____

_____

_____

_____

_____

Snacks:_____

_____

Comments:_____

_____

_____

_____

PRIMAL LIFESTYLE   Success Score:_____

Sleep (1-10):_____   Comments:_____

Sun (1-10):_____   Comments:_____

Play (1-10):_____   Comments:_____

Brain (1-10):_____   Comments:_____

Move (1-10):_____   Comments:_____

PERSONAL

Comments:_____

_____

_____

_____

EXERCISE   Success Score:_____   Effort Score:_____

Workout:_____

Location:_____   Duration:_____

Exercise 1:_____ Weight:_____ Reps/Time:_____ Set 2:_____ Set 3:_____

Exercise 2:_____ Weight:_____ Reps/Time:_____ Set 2:_____ Set 3:_____

Exercise 3:_____ Weight:_____ Reps/Time:_____ Set 2:_____ Set 3:_____

Exercise 4:_____ Weight:_____ Reps/Time:_____ Set 2:_____ Set 3:_____

Exercise 5:_____ Weight:_____ Reps/Time:_____ Set 2:_____ Set 3:_____

Exercise 6:_____ Weight:_____ Reps/Time:_____ Set 2:_____ Set 3:_____

Comments:_____

_____

_____

_____

_____

Workout:_____

Location:_____ Distance:_____ Duration:_____

Comments:_____

_____

_____

_____

_____

SUMMARY

Tomorrow:_____

This Week:_____ This Month:_____

Wins:_____

Challenges:_____

Comments:_____

_____

_____

_____

_____

_____

One Word   Success Score (1-10)

DAY 90 EVALUATION

/ / DATE

DIET   Past 90 days.

Success Score:_____

Wins:_____

Challenges:_____

Comments:_____

_____

_____

_____

_____

1 - 10 SCORE

Energy:	"Big M":	Health:	Mood:	Stress:

MACRONUTRIENT CALCULATIONS

Carbs:	Protein:	Fat:	Calories:

PRIMAL LIFESTYLE   Past 90 days.

Success Score:_____

Sleep (1-10):_____   Comments:_____

Sun (1-10):_____   Comments:_____

Play (1-10):_____   Comments:_____

Brain (1-10):_____   Comments:_____

Move (1-10):_____   Comments:_____

PERSONAL   Past 90 days.

Comments:_____

_____

_____

_____

_____

_____

_____

_____

DAY 90 EVALUATION

EXERCISE   Past 30 days.

Success Score:_____   Effort Score:_____

Wins:_____

Challenges:_____

Comments:_____

_____

_____

_____

GOALS

1._____

2._____

3._____

4._____

5._____

BODY MEASUREMENTS

Time of Day:_____   Scale/method used:_____

Day 1 weight:_____   Day 1 fat %:_____

Day 2 weight:_____   Day 2 fat %:_____

Day 3 weight:_____   Day 3 fat %:_____

Average weight:_____   Average body fat %:_____

Body part measurements:.

Waistline:_____ Hips:_____ Chest:_____

Thighs:_____ Biceps:_____

Other body measurement:_____ Value:_____

Other body measurement:_____ Value:_____

DAY 90 EVALUATION

FITNESS MEASUREMENTS

Morning resting heart rate:_____   _____   _____   Average:_____
                              Day 1   Day 2   Day 3

Primal Essential Movements – one set maximum effort

Note type of progression or advanced exercise if not actual Essential Movement
(e.g. – decline pushups, chair-assisted pullups)

Pushups:_____ Number:_____

Pullups:_____ Number:_____

Squats:_____ Number:_____

Plank:_____ Time:_____

400-meter run:_____   Date:_____

Location/conditions/notes:_____

One-mile run:_____   Date:_____

Location/conditions/notes:_____

_____

Maximum Aerobic Function test

Date:_____ Heart Rate:_____

Course/distance:_____ Time:_____

Location/conditions/notes:_____

VO2 Max test (ml/kg value):_____

Date/location/method of test: _____

Other best performances:

Event/Exercise:_____ Achievement:_____

Event/Exercise:_____ Achievement:_____

Event/Exercise:_____ Achievement:_____

```
┌ ─ ─ ─ ─ ─ ─ ─ ─ ─ ─ ─ ─ ─ ─ ─ ─ ─ ┐
│                                   │
│                                   │
│                                   │
│                                   │
│                                   │
│          Affix "After" photo here.│
│                                   │
│                                   │
│                                   │
│                                   │
│                                   │
│                                   │
└ ─ ─ ─ ─ ─ ─ ─ ─ ─ ─ ─ ─ ─ ─ ─ ─ ─ ┘
```

Comments on "After" photo:_____

_____

How does your "After" photo compare to your "Before" photo?:

_____

_____

_____

What specific differences did you notice?:

_____

_____

_____

Rate your satisfaction with the "Before/After" photo changes on a scale of 1–10:_____

BASELINE BLOOD VALUES

BLOOD CHEMESTRY

Blood pressure:_____ / _____   _____ / _____   _____ / _____
             Day 1   Day 2   Day 3

Average blood pressure:_____ / _____

CBC markers:

Hematocrit %:_____

Iron marker_____   Number:_____

White blood cells:_____   25-vitamin D (ng/ml):_____

Fasting blood insulin:_____   HbA1C (average blood glucose):_____

Plasma viscosity:_____   Glutamine _____

Other CBC Marker:_____   Number:_____ Avg range:_____

Other CBC Marker:_____   Number:_____ Avg range:_____

Other CBC Marker:_____   Number:_____ Avg range:_____

INFLAMMATION MARKERS

hs-CRP:_____   IL-6:_____   Lp2A:_____

Homocysteine:_____   Creatine phosphokinase (CPK):_____

Omega-3 marker #1:_____   Number:_____

Omega-3 marker #2:_____   Number:_____

Other inflammation #1:_____   Number:_____ Avg range:_____

Other inflammation #2:_____   Number:_____ Avg range:_____

Other inflammation #3:_____   Number:_____ Avg range:_____

BASELINE BLOOD VALUES

LIPIDS

Apolipoprotein B (ApoB):_____   Triglyceride/HDL ratio:_____

Total cholesterol:_____   HDL:_____   LDL:_____

Triglycerides:_____

Total cholesterol/HDL ratio:_____

Lipid marker #1:_____   Number:_____

Lipid marker #2:_____   Number:_____

HORMONES

Testosterone marker:_____   Number:_____

Cortisol (serum):_____   Cortisol (salivary):_____

Thyroid marker:_____   Number:_____

Melatonin:_____

Hormone marker #1:_____   Number:_____   Normal range:_____

Hormone marker #2:_____   Number:_____   Normal range:_____

Hormone marker #3:_____   Number:_____   Normal range:_____

CANCER SCREENINGS

CEA (colon):_____   CA 125 (ovarian):_____   CA 27.29 (breast):_____

AFB blood test:_____   PSA (prostate):_____

URINALYSIS

Marker #1:_____   Number:_____   Average range:_____

Marker #2:_____   Number:_____   Average range:_____

Marker #3:_____   Number:_____   Average range:_____

DAY 90 BLOOD VALUES

BLOOD CHEMESTRY

Blood pressure:_____ / _____   _____ / _____   _____ / _____
                Day 1   Day 2   Day 3

Average blood pressure:_____ / _____

CBC markers:

Hematocrit %:_____

Iron marker_____   Number:_____

White blood cells:_____   25-vitamin D (ng/ml):_____

Fasting blood insulin:_____   HbA1C (average blood glucose):_____

Plasma viscosity:_____   Glutamine _____

Other CBC Marker:_____   Number:_____ Avg range:_____

Other CBC Marker:_____   Number:_____ Avg range:_____

Other CBC Marker:_____   Number:_____ Avg range:_____

INFLAMMATION MARKERS

hs-CRP:_____   IL-6:_____   Lp2A:_____

Homocysteine:_____   Creatine phosphokinase (CPK):_____

Omega-3 marker #1:_____   Number:_____

Omega-3 marker #2:_____   Number:_____

Other inflammation #1:_____   Number:_____ Avg range:_____

Other inflammation #2:_____   Number:_____ Avg range:_____

Other inflammation #3:_____   Number:_____ Avg range:_____

DAY 90 BLOOD VALUES

LIPIDS

Apolipoprotein B (ApoB):_____   Triglyceride/HDL ratio:_____

Total cholesterol:_____   HDL:_____   LDL:_____

Triglycerides:_____

Total cholesterol/HDL ratio:_____

Lipid marker #1:_____   Number:_____

Lipid marker #2:_____   Number:_____

HORMONES

Testosterone marker:_____   Number:_____

Cortisol (serum):_____   Cortisol (salivary):_____

Thyroid marker:_____   Number:_____

Melatonin:_____

Hormone marker #1:_____   Number:_____   Normal range:_____

Hormone marker #2:_____   Number:_____   Normal range:_____

Hormone marker #3:_____   Number:_____   Normal range:_____

CANCER SCREENINGS

CEA (colon):_____   CA 125 (ovarian):_____   CA 27.29 (breast):_____

AFB blood test:_____   PSA (prostate):_____

URINALYSIS

Marker #1:_____   Number:_____   Average range:_____

Marker #2:_____   Number:_____   Average range:_____

Marker #3:_____   Number:_____   Average range:_____

RESOURCES

21-DAY TRANSFORMATION KEY CONCEPTS AND ACTION ITEMS

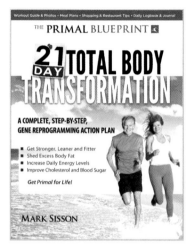

Understanding the Primal Blueprint philosophy and implementing these lifestyle practices can be a tall order, particularly when you've been socialized your entire life by Conventional Wisdom to do something different – or even in direct opposition to – Primal practices. In the three years after the initial publication of *The Primal Blueprint* hardcover book, my staff and I have received tons of feedback from readers, MarksDailyApple.com visitors, and guests at our nationwide series of Primal seminars. Certain patterns have emerged from the feedback we've analyzed. People seem to get stuck in the same areas – having trouble understanding, agreeing with, or implementing certain elements of the Primal approach. This feedback helps illuminate the most important element of the message for followers to "own".

Consequently, I crafted what I feel are the eight most relevant Key Concepts to understand about the Primal Blueprint, following by the five most impactful Action Items that will kick-start a Primal lifestyle. These topics frame the content of my 2011 guidebook called *The Primal Blueprint 21-Day Total Body Transformation*. This book – filled with photos, practical tips, and a 21-day step-by-step program to implement the Action Items, is a great way to cut to the chase of what Primal living is all about. For our purposes in the 90-Day Journal, I have briefly summarized the eight Key Concepts and five Action Items that comprise the 21-Day book. With an understanding of the Key Concepts, you can implement the five Action Items with confidence and smoothly transition into a custom-designed Primal lifestyle – dialing in your eating, exercise, sleep, and play for the rest of your life.

KEY CONCEPTS

1. YES, YOU REALLY CAN REPROGRAM YOUR GENES: More than just determining your fixed heritable traits, genes are responsible for continually directing the production of the proteins that control how your body functions every second. Genes turn on or off only in response to signals they receive from the environment surrounding them – signals that you provide based on the foods you eat, the types of exercise you do (or don't do), your sleeping habits, sun exposure and so forth.

2. THE CLUES TO OPTIMAL GENE EXPRESSION ARE FOUND IN EVOLUTION: Two million years of selection pressure and harsh environmental circumstances created the perfect genetic recipe for human health and longevity. Our genes expect us to be lean, fit and healthy by modeling the lifestyle behaviors and diets of our hunter-gatherer ancestors even in the context of hectic modern life. Plants and animals (meat/fish/fowl/eggs, vegetables, fruits, nuts and seeds) should comprise the entirety of the human diet, with allowances for the moderate intake of certain modern foods. As for exercise forms and frequency, less is often more.

3. YOUR BODY PREFERS BURNING FAT OVER CARBOHYDRATES: Conventional Wisdom's grain-based, low-fat diet has artificially created a sugar and carbohydrate-based metabolism that you've been stuck in, and suffering from, for your entire life. Going Primal shifts you into the fat-based, all-day energy metabolism that has supported human survival for two million years. This is the most liberating aspect of Primal living.

4. 80 PERCENT OF YOUR BODY COMPOSITION SUCCESS IS DETERMINED BY HOW YOU EAT: Many modern foods (even ones you thought were healthy) are causing you to gain weight and get sick. Moderating insulin production by ditching grains, sugars and legumes, and lowering inflammation by eliminating harmful manmade fats, will promote efficient reduction of excess body fat, effortless maintenance of ideal body composition, increased daily energy levels, decreased risk of illness, and optimal function of various other hormonal systems (stress, appetite, immune, metabolic, sleep, thyroid, etc.).

5. GRAINS ARE TOTALLY UNNECESSARY: The centerpiece of the Standard American Diet (SAD), grains – even whole grains – offer minimal nutritional value, promote fat storage by raising insulin, and contain anti-nutrients that promote inflammation, compromise digestion, and often interfere with immune function. There is no good reason to make grains (or legumes, for that matter) any part of your diet unless you want a cheap source of calories that easily convert to sugar.

6. SATURATED FAT AND CHOLESTEROL ARE NOT YOUR ENEMY: The Conventional Wisdom story about heart disease is only validated when you wash high fat foods down with a ton of grains and sugars. Cholesterol is one of the body's most vital molecules. Saturated fat is our preferred fuel. The true heart disease risk factors – oxidation and inflammation – are driven strongly by polyunsaturated fats, simple sugars, excess insulin production and stress. Limiting processed carbohydrates and eating more high quality fats and whole foods (including saturated animal fat) can promote health, weight management, and reduced risk of heart disease.

7. EXERCISE IS INEFFECTIVE FOR WEIGHT MANAGEMENT: Burning calories through exercise has little influence on your ability to achieve and maintain ideal body composition. When you depend on carbohydrate (glucose) as your primary fuel, exercise simply stimulates increased appetite and calorie intake. Chronic exercise patterns inhibit fat metabolism, break down lean muscle tissue, and lead to fatigue, injury, and burnout.

8. MAXIMUM FITNESS CAN BE ACHIEVED IN MINIMAL TIME WITH HIGH INTENSITY WORKOUTS: Regular brief, intense strength training sessions and occasional all-out sprints promote optimal gene expression and broad athletic competency. Enjoy more benefits in a fraction of the time spent doing the chronic exercise advocated by Conventional Wisdom.

ACTION ITEMS

1. ELIMINATE SAD FOODS: Out with the objectionable foods that promote weight gain and chronic health problems: Sugars, grains, processed fats, packaged snacks, etc.

2. SHOP, COOK, AND DINE PRIMALLY: Re-stock your pantry and kitchen with Primal foods, and implement winning strategies for shopping, meal preparation, dining out, and snacking.

3. MAKE THE HEALTHIEST CHOICES ACROSS THE SPECTRUM: Meat, fish, fowl, eggs, vegetables, fruits, nuts and seeds, fats and oils, foods allowed in moderation such as dairy, and occasional sensible indulgences.

4. EXERCISE PRIMALLY: MOVE, LIFT, AND SPRINT!: Pursue broad athletic competency with an intuitive blend of workouts honoring the three Primal Blueprint Fitness laws (Move Frequently at a Slow Pace, Lift Heavy Things, and Sprint Once in a While).

5. SLOW LIFE DOWN: Take the time to enjoy simple pleasures such as "slow food" over industrialized food; balanced instead of chronic exercise; focused work habits instead of multitasking; interpersonal relationships over social media; calm, relaxing evenings instead of excessive artificial light and digital stimulation; and plenty of time for play, sun exposure, rest and relaxation.

PRIMAL BLUEPRINT FOOD PYRAMID

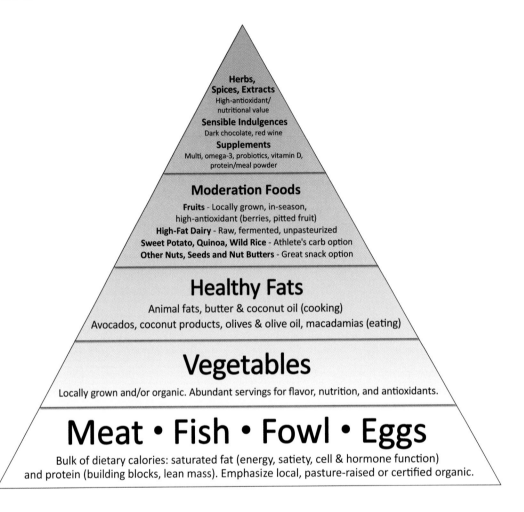

Herbs, Spices, Extracts
High-antioxidant/ nutritional value
Sensible Indulgences
Dark chocolate, red wine
Supplements
Multi, omega-3, probiotics, vitamin D, protein/meal powder

Moderation Foods
Fruits - Locally grown, in-season, high-antioxidant (berries, pitted fruit)
High-Fat Dairy - Raw, fermented, unpasteurized
Sweet Potato, Quinoa, Wild Rice - Athlete's carb option
Other Nuts, Seeds and Nut Butters - Great snack option

Healthy Fats
Animal fats, butter & coconut oil (cooking)
Avocados, coconut products, olives & olive oil, macadamias (eating)

Vegetables
Locally grown and/or organic. Abundant servings for flavor, nutrition, and antioxidants.

Meat • Fish • Fowl • Eggs
Bulk of dietary calories: saturated fat (energy, satiety, cell & hormone function) and protein (building blocks, lean mass). Emphasize local, pasture-raised or certified organic.

PYRAMID NOTES: The Primal Blueprint Food Pyramid conveys which foods and categories to emphasize in the model of our hunter-gatherer ancestors. Meal emphasis should be on vegetables; think heaping portions crowding the plate, instead of the small-serving accoutrements we are accustomed to. However, most of your calories will come from animal foods (meat, fish, fowl and eggs) due to their caloric density. Notice the distinction to be selective with fruit as well as nuts and seeds. High fruit consumption, particularly year-round, can compromise weight loss efforts. Nuts and seeds, while excellent sources of nutrition, have unfavorable O6:O3 ratios, something of increasing concern to Primal enthusiasts. Macadamia's earn special distinction since they are 84 percent monounsaturated and have minimal significance to omega-6:omega-3 dietary ratios.

PRIMAL BLUEPRINT CARBOHYDRATE CURVE

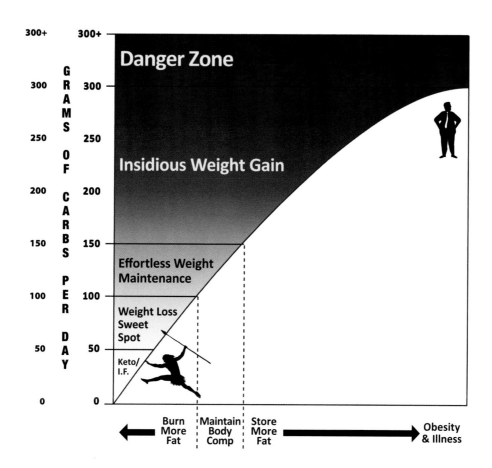

The curve illustrates how various levels of average daily carbohydrate intake impact your health and weight management. Moderating the wildly excessive carbohydrate intake from the Standard American Diet down to genetically optimal levels is your key to weight loss success, and avoiding today's prevalent diet-related health problems and disease.

0 to 50 grams per day: *Ketosis and Accelerated Fat Burning*
Excellent catalyst for quick reduction of excess body fat through Intermittent Fasting or devoted carb restriction.

50 to 100 grams per day: *Primal Sweet Spot for Effortless Weight Loss* Minimizes insulin production and accelerates fat metabolism. Supports abundant intake of vegetables, reasonable intake of seasonal fruits, nuts, and seeds, and occasional indulgences. Enables steady reduction of excess body fat (4-8 pounds per month; 1.8-3.6 kilos) with no deprivation.

100 to 150 grams per day: *Primal Blueprint Maintenance Range* Allows for genetically optimal fat burning, muscle development, and effortless weight maintenance. Rationale supported by humans eating and evolving in this range or below for two million years. Dietary emphasis on animal foods and vegetables, with grains and processed sugars eliminated.

150 to 300 grams per day: *Steady, Insidious Weight Gain* Continuous insulin-stimulating effects inhibit fat metabolism and contribute to widespread health conditions. The de facto recommendation of many popular diets and health authorities (including the USDA Food Pyramid!) and easy to default into when grains are a dietary centerpiece.

300 or more grams per day: *Danger Zone!* Zone of the average American's diet, based on grains and with soda and other sugars added on. Promotes Metabolic Syndrome, type 2 diabetes, obesity, and numerous other significant health problems. Immediate and dramatic reduction of grains, sugars, sweetened beverages and other processed carbs is critical.

Carb Curve Variables: The 50-gram/200-calorie range within each zone on the curve allows for individual disparities in body weight and metabolic rate (e.g. - small female – low end; large male – upper end). Athletes or other mega-calorie burners can adjust curve values upward by perhaps 100 grams of carbs per hour of vigorous exercise. This will ensure proper fueling for and recovery from workouts, and likely support effortless weight maintenance. Keep in mind that the curve values represent averages over the long-term. Relax, enjoy Primal-approved meals, and don't obsess about macronutrient breakdowns at each meal.

PRIMAL ESSENTIAL MEALS

Eating Primally doesn't have to be complex or time-consuming. Many people transitioning away from long-standing dietary habits find success comes easily when they repeat a pattern of their favorite Primal-approved meals. Here's a quick look at how a day of Primal eating might look, with details provided in *The Primal Blueprint 21-Day Total Body Transformation*.

BREAKFAST

Primal Omelet: 3-5 pasture-raised or organic eggs, butter, chopped vegetables, chopped bacon or other meat, seasonings. Saute vegetables separately, and cook meat separately. Pour whisked eggs into buttered skillet and cover over medium heat. When eggs have set, spread veggie and meat ingredients onto half of pan and carefully 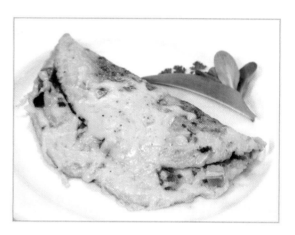 fold entire side of omelet over ingredients. Press lightly on omelet and cook until interior is no longer runny.

Primal Smoothie: ½ cup of liquid (water or coconut milk), ½ cup of ice, 2 scoops of Primal Fuel (a high protein meal replacement; any high quality whey protein supplement will also work). Optional frozen (peeled) banana or berries. Blend ingredients and serve

Other: Leftover meat and vegetables from last night's meal, a handful of macadamia nuts, or fast until lunch as you become more Primal-adapted.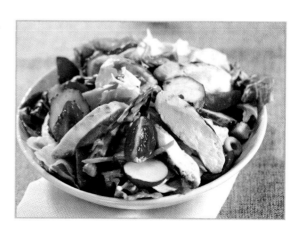

LUNCH

Primal Salad: Salad greens, chopped raw veggies (prepare large quantities and store for repeated use), chopped cooked meat (chicken, beef, salmon, tuna), chopped nuts, domestic extra-virgin olive oil dressing. Mix ingredients together and enjoy what I consider the centerpiece of Primal eating: a delicious, filling, high antioxidant, low carbohydrate midday meal!

Primal Wrap: Use a large leaf of iceberg lettuce to serve as your "bread", and apply your favorite sandwich ingredients: tuna salad, BLT, turkey Cobb, etc.

DINNER

Primal Meat and Vegetables: Fry or grill your favorite meat (steak, lamb, pork, bison, chicken, turkey or fish). Accompany with some steamed or pan-fried (liberally in butter or coconut oil) vegetables (onions, peppers, mushrooms, asparagus, broccoli, leafy greens, etc.). Simple. Easy to prepare. Delicious!

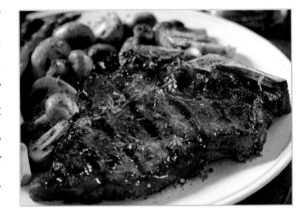

SNACKS

Surround yourself with Primal snacks to make your transition easy and convenient: Berries, dark chocolate (75 percent cacao content or higher), canned fish (herring, mackerel, sardines, tuna), hard-boiled eggs, jerky, macadamia nuts, olives, trail mix, raw vegetables (great with nut butter).

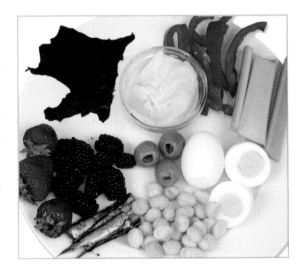

PRIMAL FOODS - BEST TO WORST SPECTRUM

MEAT, FOWL, AND EGGS

1. Local, pasture-raised: Superior omega-3 and nutrient values due to natural diet of grass, insects, etc.

2. USDA-certified organic: Likely grain-fed but free of objectionable hormones, pesticides, and antibiotics.

3. Humane-raised, hormone-free, grass-finished or other distinctive labeling: Terminologies are loosely-regulated and not entirely helpful, but efforts to distinguish as other than conventional CAFO meat are worth recognizing.

4. Conventional CAFO: Animals raised in Concentrated Animal Feeding Operations typically contain hormones (to promote faster growth and increase profits), pesticides (ingested from inferior feed sources), and antibiotics (to prevent infection from living in cramped, dirty quarters). CAFO products are nutritionally inferior to pasture-raised or organic animals. If you must eat CAFO products, trim the fat before cooking to limit exposure to toxins.

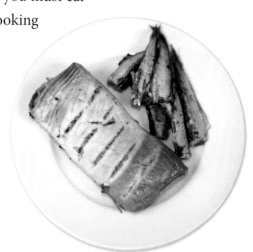

FISH - RANKED

1. Wild-caught, oily, cold water fish from remote, pollution-free waters: Highest omega-3 values of any food (salmon, sardines, herring, mackerel, anchovies).

2. Other wild-caught fish: Stick with domestic sources such as trout.

3. Approved farmed fish: Domestic coho salmon, shellfish, barramundi, catfish, crayfish, tilapia, and trout are acceptable.

FISH - AVOID

1. Most farmed fish: High levels of chemical contaminants, unsanitary waters, poor omega-6:omega-3 ratios, and overall significantly lower nutritional value than wild-caught fish. Includes Atlantic salmon, by far the most common type of salmon sold – with an estimated 90% of the market share.

2. Top of food chain: Avoid sword and shark due to high concentrations of mercury and other contaminants.

3. Asian imports: Avoid both farmed and wild-caught fish imported from China and other Asian countries, due to minimal safety regulations and polluted waters.

4. Visit montereybayaquarium.org or edf.com for further guidelines on eating healthy, sustainable fish and avoiding objectionable fish.

VEGETABLES

1. Locally-grown, pesticide-free: Superior nutritional and antioxidant value. Enjoy heaping portions!

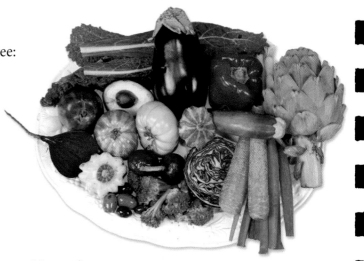

2. USDA-certified organic: Local actually ranks above organic for sustainability and optimal growing and ripening conditions.

3. Conventionally grown: Thoroughly wash conventionally grown veggies with soft, edible skin (leafy greens, peppers).

4. Remote, conventionally grown: Strive to do better, but by no means objectionable in the big picture.

FRUITS

1. Locally-grown, pesticide-free, in-season: Enjoy liberal servings as Grok did. If you are trying to lose excess body fat, selectivity and moderation are warranted. High antioxidant, low glycemic are best, including all berries, most stone (pitted) fruits (cherries, prunes, peaches, apricots), avocado, casaba melon, lime, lemon, tomato, and guava.

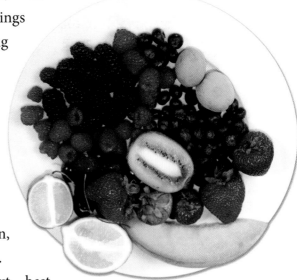

2. USDA-certified organic: Next best choice. Try to find fruits grown closer to home and emphasize them during natural ripening season.

3. Conventionally grown: Wash fruits with soft, edible skin thoroughly.

4. High glycemic, low antioxidant: Moderate intake or avoid due to inferior nutritional value/body fat concerns: dates, dried fruits (all), grapes, mangoes, melons, nectarines, oranges, papayas, pineapples, plums, and tangerines.

5. Remote, conventionally grown, out of season. Probably not a necessary component of a healthy diet, especially if you are trying to lose excess body fat.

FATS AND OILS - APPROVED

1. Avocado, Olives/Olive Oil: Excellent monounsaturated fat sources. For olive oil, find domestic sources of extra-virgin, first cold-press only; superior to more common imported, over-processed products.

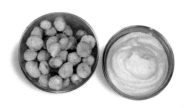

2. Coconut products: Oil, milk, butter, water, flakes and other derivatives provide numerous health

benefits, including difficult to obtain medium-chain fatty acids. Convenient replacement for objectionable milk, flour, and PUFA products.

3. Cooking fats: Butter, coconut oil, other saturated animal fats. Saturated fats are temperature stable, so they won't oxidize under high heat as PUFAs do.

4. High omega-3 oils: Borage, cod liver, krill, hemp, salmon – easier to assimilate than the more common flax seed oil. Marine oil – commonly used in gel capsules.

5. Macadamia nuts: Earn special distinction above other nuts and seeds due to less objectionable omega-6:omega-3 ratios, high monounsaturated fat content and superior nutritional and antioxidant values. Enjoy liberally as a go-to Primal snack. Try macadamia nut butter for a delicious veggie spread or dessert treat on dark chocolate!

FATS AND OILS – AVOID

1. PUFA (polyunsaturated fatty acids): Canola, corn, soybean, safflower, sunflower and other vegetable and seed oils, margarine, shortening. Easily oxidized and promoting pro-inflammatory condition in the body. Switch to saturated animal fats.

2. Trans and partially-hydrogenated oils: Found in a variety of packaged, frozen and processed foods. Causes destruction at the cellular level; total elimination is critical.

MODERATION FOODS

1. Beverages: Hydrate using thirst as guideline; reject unfounded Conventional Wisdom promoting habitual over-drinking. Coffee is acceptable in moderation;

refrain from using as an energy crutch or stick with decaf. Club soda or mineral water with lemon, lime, and salt pinch added can give a fizzy fix to those kicking soda habits. Green or herbal teas offer anti-inflammatory and immune supporting benefits.

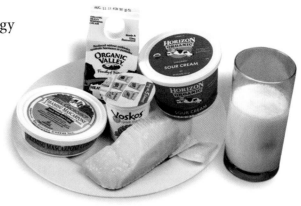

2. High fat dairy products: Raw, fermented, unpasteurized, unsweetened is best (ghee, butter, cream, cheese, cottage cheese, Greek yogurt, kefir, raw whole milk). Try to find pasture-raised/grass-fed.

3. Other nuts, seeds and their derivative butters: Excellent nutritional value, but some moderation warranted due to concerns about omega-6:omega-3 imbalances in the modern diet. Walnuts, almonds, and pumpkin seeds have great nutritional value.

4. Supplemental carbs: High calorie burners without excess body fat concerns can enjoy sweet potatoes, quinoa, and wild rice to restock glycogen after heavy exercise. Others might consider these carbs "indulgences" – not necessary for health or exercise recovery when Primal-adapted.

SENSIBLE INDULGENCES

1. Dark chocolate: Superior option to satisfy your sweet tooth; high antioxidant, high fat satisfaction. Go for 75 percent cacao content or higher.

2. Red wine: Best alcohol choice due to excellent antioxidant benefits. Note alcohol calories are burned first, putting fat loss on hold while you indulge. Enjoy responsibly and in moderation.

PRIMAL BLUEPRINT FITNESS PYRAMID

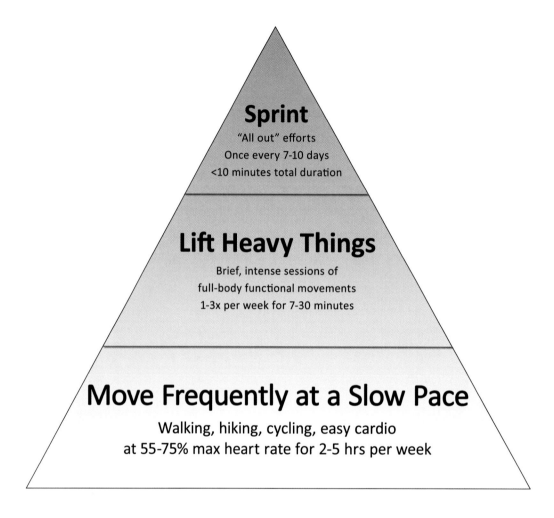

Sprint
"All out" efforts
Once every 7-10 days
<10 minutes total duration

Lift Heavy Things
Brief, intense sessions of
full-body functional movements
1-3x per week for 7-30 minutes

Move Frequently at a Slow Pace
Walking, hiking, cycling, easy cardio
at 55-75% max heart rate for 2-5 hrs per week

PYRAMID NOTES: The pyramid reflects the exercise patterns that shaped human evolution for 2.5 million years. Becoming fit, or even super fit, does not have to involve a complex, time-consuming approach. All you have to do is engage in a sensible blend of Primal workouts, which are scalable to people of all fitness levels.

The "Move Frequently" goal involves structured aerobic workouts and finding various ways to move more in everyday life. For "Lift Heavy Things", you can enjoy great benefits from a workout as short as seven minutes – really! Even advanced exercisers need not continue for more than 30 minutes very often, and never over 60. Brief and intense is the key to stimulate the flow of adaptive hormones and prevent chronic exercise patterns.

HEART RATE CALCULATIONS

TRAINING RANGES

Below 55 percent of maximum: Insufficient to be considered a "workout". For most people this is a slow walk.

55-75 percent of maximum: Optimal range for aerobic exercise. Pace is comfortable enough to allow you to converse during exercise, and feel refreshed (instead of worn out) afterward. For the unfit, 75 percent can be reached by briskly walking, or easy cruising on the bike or cardio machines. Fit people can jog or move at a steady pace on bicycle or cardio machine and remain at or below 75 percent.

75-85 percent of maximum: We might call this "No man's land"! Not strenuous enough to be considered high-intensity Primal exercise, but too difficult to deliver optimal aerobic benefits. Frequent sustained exercise in this zone – unfortunately the default zone for many gymgoers and endurance athletes – can lead to a destructive "Chronic Cardio" training pattern. Occasional brisk workouts in this zone are acceptable and beneficial when balanced with adequate rest and low intensity workouts.

85-100 percent of maximum: Zone of high intensity workouts such as sprinting, strenuous group classes, or competitive sports. Best results come from infrequent efforts lasting 30 minutes or less.

"The reason I'll never go back to living any other way in one word: bacon."

– Success Story Lindsay

PRIMAL ESSENTIAL MOVEMENTS

The Primal Essential Movements (PEM) promote full body, functional fitness with exercises that are simple, safe, and scalable to all fitness levels through a series of easier progression exercises. Warmup and cooldown at each session with a few minutes of easy cardio. Conduct an assessment (one set, maximum effort) to determine your starting point exercise. The goal is to reach the male and female mastery level listed with each exercise, then move up to the next progression exercise. Advanced exercisers can don a weighted vest to add degree of difficulty, or review more options in the *Primal Blueprint Fitness* eBook available at MarksDailyApple.com.

PUSHUPS

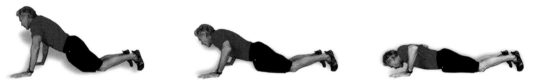

Easiest - Knee Pushup: male 50, female 30. Do pushups on the ground, but assuming a plank position on your knees.

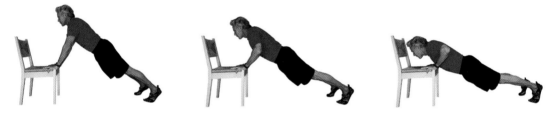

Next - Incline Pushup: male 50, female 25. Do pushups with hands resting on a bench or other object elevated from ground.

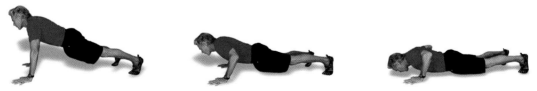

Baseline Pushups: Plank position, arms extended, shoulder width, hands forward. Lower to ground – chest touching first! Keep body dead straight, core and glutes tight, head and neck neutral to torso. Elbows bend backwards at 45-degree angle.

Baseline Essential Movement Mastery: male 50, female 20.

PULL-UPS

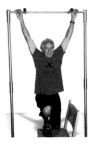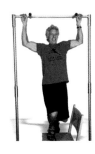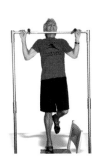

Easiest - Chair-Assisted Pullup: male 20, female 15.

Emphasize upper body muscles and use just enough leg force to help get your chin over the bar for the appropriate number of reps.

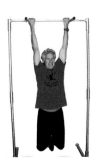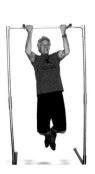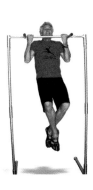

Next - Chin Up (inverted grip): male 7, female 4.

May be slightly easier than overhand grip, particularly if you have wrist, elbow, or shoulder issues.

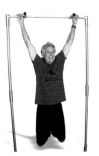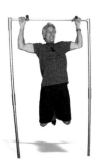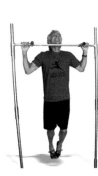

Baseline Pullups (overhand grip): Baseline Pullup: Elbows tight, chin tucked, shoulder blades pinched, lower body quiet. Lead with chest, raise chin over bar, and lower until arms extend.

Baseline Essential Movement Mastery: male 12, female 5.

SQUATS

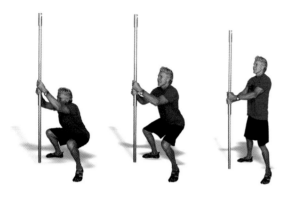

Easiest - Assisted Squat: male 50, female 50.

Hold pole or support object while lowering into and raising up from squat position. Use support object as little as possible.

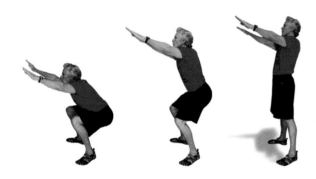

Baseline Squats: Feet shoulder-width or slightly wider. Toes forward or naturally pointed outward slightly. Lower yourself by extending your butt out and bringing thighs to just below parallel to the ground. Stand back up completely, making sure your knees track in line with your feet.

Baseline Essential Movement Mastery: male 50, female 50.

PLANKS

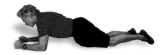

Easiest - Forearm/Knee Plank: male and female two minutes. Assume plank position with forearms and knees resting on ground. Tense core and glutes during exercise.

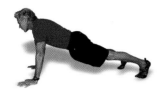

Next - Hand/Feet Plank: male and female two minutes. Assume plank position a la pushup starting point, with hands and feet on ground.

Baseline Elbow/Feet Plank:

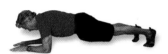

Elbows on ground, aligned with shoulders. Raise onto toes with body horizontal. Tuck tailbone a bit to alleviate potential back stress. You can add difficulty by moving to side plank position to isolate lateral ab muscles. Face body sideways in straight head-to-toe position (don't sag the hips!), holding for 45 seconds each side.

PEM ISOLATION

For a unique challenge, set an ambitious numerical goal for a single PEM exercise and make that your entire workout one day. Perform reps until failure, then rest as needed and tackle additional reps, counting your accumulated total to reach your goal. For example, some mornings I'll aspire to do 200 decline pushups. These might accumulate in sets as follows: 60, 30, 50, 25, 25, and 15, with rest periods between the sets ranging from 30 seconds to three minutes.

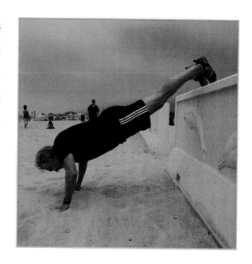

PRIMAL SPRINT WORKOUTS

Find a location with 50-100 meters of smooth ground. You can also sprint on a stationary bike or other cardio machines for a no impact sprint workout. Obtain medical clearance before conducting intense workouts, such as those described in this book. Begin each workout with a five-minute warmup of low intensity walking or jogging (55-75 percent of maximum heart rate) followed by sequence of dynamic stretching and technique drills as pictured in the 21-Day book. Conclude each workout with a five minute cool down identical to the warmup.

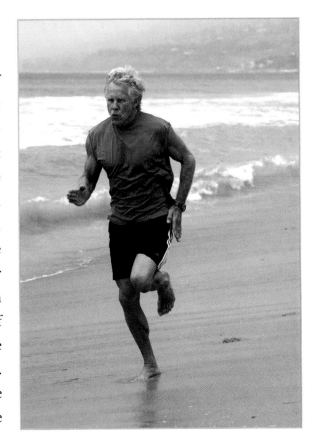

BASIC SPRINT WORKOUT - STRIDES AND SPRINTS

Six times warmup "strides" of 8-15 seconds each (65-75 percent of max effort), with a 20 second rest period between strides. Then, six times 8-15 second sprints at 75-85 percent of max effort. Rest one minute, or otherwise enough to breathe normally before next effort. Use a moving, gradual start into each sprint.

As your conditioning improves, increase sprinting effort up to 100 percent. Keep the set of strides as a warmup at 65-75 percent, where form is the main focus. For a lower impact option, conduct this workout on an uphill grade; walk or jog back down to starting point for recovery.

SPRINT WORKOUT #2 - ACCELERATIONS

Six to eight times 30-second sprints with the first ten seconds at medium effort, second ten seconds at hard effort and third ten seconds at full sprint. One to two minutes recovery between efforts to achieve normal respiration.

SPRINT WORKOUT #3 - TECHNIQUE DRILLS

- **Strides:** Four times eight-second strides at 75 percent effort. Ten seconds rest between efforts. One minute rest before next exercise.
- **Skipping:** Two to four times 50 meters. Take off on left leg while driving right knee as high as you can (try to hit your chest). Land on left leg, then take off on right leg while driving left knee to your chest – like an exaggerated skip. Strive for maximum height instead of length. Fifteen seconds rest between efforts. One minute rest before next exercise.
- **Bounding:** Two to four times 50 meters. Take as long a stride as possible, focusing on keeping your balance rather than speed. Thirty seconds rest between efforts. One minute rest before next exercise.
- **Bunny Hopping:** Two to four times 50 meters. Take off on both legs and jump up and forward. Focus on achieving a good balance between height and length. Swing arms to assist effort and ensure a balanced landing. Lower into squat position, with thighs parallel to ground, to initiate each hop. One minute rest between efforts (you'll need it, trust me). Two minutes rest before next exercise.
- **Full Sprint:** Two to four times 50 meter full sprint. One minute rest between efforts.

SPRINT WORKOUT #4 - PEM / SPRINT COMBO

This is a fun session that's over with quickly and integrates strength training and sprinting. It's a great challenge for all of your muscle groups and your cardiovascular system.

- One set maximum effort pushups, then immediately sprint 80 meters. Rest 30-60 seconds.
- One set maximum effort plank, then bunny hop 40 meters. Rest 30-60 seconds.
- One set maximum effort pull-ups, then sprint 80 meters. Rest 30-60 seconds.
- One set maximum effort squats, then bunny hop 40 meters (wow!).

CYCLING SPRINT WORKOUT #1 - INTERVAL LADDER.

Five-minute warmup pedaling at 55-75 percent of maximum heart rate. Sprint 15 seconds, rest 15 seconds. Then a 30 second sprint with 30 seconds rest. Then 45 second sprint, 45 second rest. Then 60 second sprint, 60 seconds rest. After the 60 second effort, sprint: 45, rest: 45; sprint: 30, rest: 30; sprint: 15, rest: 15 – to complete the ladder workout. Five minutes easy pedaling cool down.

CYCLING SPRINT WORKOUT #2 - TABATA INTERVALS.

Tabata is a workout system where you achieve four minutes of intense effort in sprinting, weight lifting or any other exercise, using the consistent work/rest ratio of 20 seconds sprint, 10 seconds rest, 20 seconds sprint, 10 seconds rest – repeated for four minutes. Five minutes easy pedaling cool down.

"I didn't have a scale to weigh that old fluffy mommy, but I dropped all the way down to my current 151 pounds and I'm seeing muscles that I thought were lost forever!"

– Success Story Malika

PRIMAL APPROVED
At a Glance

DIET

Beverages: Water (obey thirst), coffee, unsweetened tea.

Coconut Products: Butter, flakes, flour, milk, oil; great medium-chain fats!

Dairy: Raw, fermented, high-fat, organic (cheese, cottage cheese, cream cheese, kefir, whole milk, yogurt).

Eggs: Local, pasture-raised, or certified organic. High omega-3!

Fats & Oils: Domestic extra-virgin olive oil (eating); butter or coconut oil (cooking); fish oil (supplements).

Fish: Small, oily, wild-caught fish (anchovies, herring, mackerel, salmon, sardines); approved domestic farmed fish (coho salmon, trout, shellfish).

Fruit: Locally-grown, organic, in-season preferred. High glycemic/low antioxidant (berries, stone fruits).

Herbs and Spices: High-antioxidant, anti-inflammatory, immune-supporting, flavor-enhancing.

Indulgences: Enjoy dark chocolate (75%+ cacao content), and red wine in moderation; high antioxidant!

Macadamia Nuts: High monounsaturated, low O6; ultimate Primal snack!

Meat & Fowl: Emphasize local, pasture-raised, or USDA-certified organic.

Other Nuts, Seeds and Their Derivative Butters: Great snack option; moderate intake for O6:O3 concerns.

Snacks: Berries, canned fish, veggies and cream cheese/nut butter, hard-boiled eggs, fresh jerky, macadamia nuts, olives, seeds, trail mix.

Supplemental Carbs: Sweet potatoes, quinoa, wild rice; for mega-calorie burners with optimal body fat levels.

Supplements: Multivitamin/mineral/antioxidant formula, omega-3 fish oil, probiotics, protein powder/meal replacement, vitamin D.

Vegetables: Locally grown, organic, in-season preferred; wash edible skins.

EXERCISE

Low-Level Cardio: 2-5 hours (or more) per week of walking, hiking or other structured workouts at 55-75 percent of max heart rate; increase all forms of daily movement!

Schedule: Vary workout type, frequency, intensity, and duration, always aligned with energy levels. Be spontaneous, intuitive, and playful!

Shoes: Gradually introduce barefoot or minimalist shoe time: Strengthens feet, improves technique, reduces injury risk.

Sprinting: All-out efforts lasting 8-20 seconds, once every 7-10 days when fully energized. Regular, less strenuous "wind sprint" sessions for conditioning.

Strength Training: Full-body, functional exercises – Primal Essential Movements: pushups, pull-ups, squats, planks. Brief, intense sessions of 30 minutes or less 2x/week.

Stretching: Minimal, full-body, functional stretches to transition from active to inactive: Grok Hang and Grok Squat (detailed in *The Primal Blueprint*).

LIFESTYLE/MEDICAL CARE

Play: Enjoy daily, outdoor physical fun to enhance work productivity and stress management.

Sleep: Minimize artificial light and digital stimulation after dark, consistent bed and wake times, , UV-protection yellow/orange lenses, orange bulbs, candlelight, calm transitions into and out of sleep. Awaken naturally without alarm. Nap when necessary.

Stupid Mistakes: Cultivate hyper-vigilance and risk management skills, avoid multi-tasking and overly stressful or regimented lifestyle practices. Focus on peak performance!

Sunlight: Expose large skin surface areas as long and often as possible without burning during peak solar intensity months

Use Your Brain: Try fun, creative intellectual pursuits to stay sharp and enthusiastic for all of life's challenges.

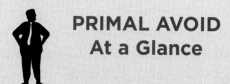

PRIMAL AVOID
At a Glance

DIET

Baking Ingredients: Flours, powders (gluten, maltodextrin, milk), starches, sweeteners (dextrose, fructose, lactose, malitol, xylitol), syrups, yeast.

Beverages: All juices (Odwalla, OJ, Ocean Spray, etc.), "energy" drinks (Red Bull, Rockstar, Monster, etc.), "milks" (almond, cow, rice, soy); powdered mixes (chai, coffee, hot chocolate); soft drinks/diet drinks; sports drinks (Gatorade, Vitamin Water); sweetened cocktails (daiquiri, eggnog, margarita); sweetened teas (Snapple, Arizona).

CAFO Meat: Moderate feedlot animals (hormones, pesticides, antibiotics, grain-feed/ high O6). Trim fat to reduce toxins. Avoid processed meats (breakfast sausage, packaged/processed dinner roasts); smoked, cured, nitrate or nitrite-treated meats (bologna, ham, hot dogs, jerky, pepperoni, salami).

Coffee: Avoid excessive use as caffeine rush. Move around or take a nap instead!

Condiments/Cooking Items: Honey mustard; jams, jellies, ketchup, mayonnaise and mayo "spreads", low-fat salad dressings, anything with high-fructose corn syrup or PUFA oils.

Dairy: Non- and low-fat (ice cream, milk, processed cheese, yogurt/frozen yogurt), conventional/GMO products (hormone, pesticide, antibiotic, allergenic, immune-suppressing).

Eggs: Limit mass produced eggs (fed with grains, hormones, pesticides and antibiotics) in favor of local, pastured eggs.

Fast Food: Chemically treated, deep fried, insulin-stimulating, devoid of nutritional value.

Fish: All Asian imports, most farmed fish (especially Atlantic salmon – 90% of market), objectionable catch methods, or top of food chain (shark, sword).

Fruit: Avoid or limit remote/conventional/off season, and conventional with soft, edible skins (berries). Moderate intake for fat loss.

Grains: Cereal, corn, pasta, rice, wheat and all derivatives (baguettes, crackers, croissants, Danishes, donuts, graham crackers, muffins, pizza, pretzels, rolls, saltines, tortillas); breakfast foods (Cream of Wheat, cereal, French toast, granola, grits, oatmeal, pancakes, waffles); chips (corn, potato, tortilla); cooking grains (amaranth, barley, bulgur, couscous, millet, rye); pretzels; puffed snacks (Cheetos, Goldfish, popcorn, rice cakes), etc. Yep, even avoid whole grains due to concerns about lectins, glutens, phytates and too much insulin!

Legumes: Alfalfa, beans, peanuts, peanut butter, peas, lentils, soybeans, and tofu. Better than grains; still unnecessary extra carbs.

Oils: Avoid trans and partially-hydrogenated; bottled PUFA oils (canola, etc.); buttery spreads and sprays; margarine; vegetable shortening; and deep fried foods.

Processed Foods: Energy bars; fast food, fruit bars and rolls; granola bars; protein bars; frozen breakfast, dinner, and dessert products; and packaged, grain/sugar-laden snack products.

Sweets/Processed Snacks: Brownies, candy/candy bars, cake, chocolate syrup, cookies, donuts, energy bars, fruit bars/rolls, granola bars, ice cream, milk chocolate/chips, pie, sugar/sweeteners (agave, artificial sweeteners, brown sugar, cane sugar, evaporated cane juice, HFCS, honey, molasses, powdered sugar, raw sugar, table sugar), sugar/chocolate coated nuts/trail mix, popsicles/frozen desserts; syrups. The less you consume, the less you'll want!

Supplements: Avoid bulk-produced supplements with additives, fillers, binders, lubricants, extruding agents, and other synthetic chemicals.

Vegetables: Limit or avoid GMO and conventional remote, especially with large surface areas/edible skins (leafy greens, peppers).

EXERCISE

Chronic Cardio: Avoid frequent sustained workouts above 75 percent of max heart rate.

Schedule: Avoid excessive workout stress with insufficient rest (compromises health, energy, and motivation levels). Consistency is not key when it comes to fitness!

Stretching: Avoid static, isolated muscle group stretches of "cold" muscles in favor of simple, brief, dynamic stretches.

MEDICAL/LIFESTYLE

Medical: Reframe Rx drug "fix it" mentality into a "prevention" mentality; Lifestyle modification first!

Sleep: Avoid excessive evening digital stimulation, morning alarms after insufficient sleep, or fighting off nap needs with caffeine.

Stupid Mistakes: Avoid multi-tasking, zoning out, or trusting that the world will keep you safe. Don't blame others for your stupid mistakes.

"Within a month of eating Primally, my lifelong symptoms of asthma disappeared, my gastric reflux abated, I dropped 15 pounds, and ceased all prescription medication."

— **Success Story Wade**

Cut these pages out for convenient use while traveling.

TRAVEL DAILY JOURNAL   DATE: ___/___/___

1 - 10 SCORE

Energy:	"Big M":	Health:	Mood:	Stress:

DIET Success score: _____

Meals: _____
_____

Comments: _____

EXERCISE Success score: _____   Effort score: _____

Workout: _____

Location: _____   Duration: _____

Exercise 1: _____ Weight/Reps: _____ Set(s): _____
Exercise 2: _____ Weight/Reps: _____ Set(s): _____
Exercise 3: _____ Weight/Reps: _____ Set(s): _____
Exercise 4: _____ Weight/Reps: _____ Set(s): _____

PRIMAL LIFESTYLE Success score: _____

Item: _____ Comments: _____
Item: _____ Comments: _____

PERSONAL

Comments: _____
_____

One word: _____   Success score: _____

TRAVEL DAILY JOURNAL   DATE: ___/___/___

1 - 10 SCORE

Energy:	"Big M":	Health:	Mood:	Stress:

DIET Success score: _____

Meals: _____
_____

Comments: _____

EXERCISE Success score: _____   Effort score: _____

Workout: _____

Location: _____   Duration: _____

Exercise 1: _____ Weight/Reps: _____ Set(s): _____
Exercise 2: _____ Weight/Reps: _____ Set(s): _____
Exercise 3: _____ Weight/Reps: _____ Set(s): _____
Exercise 4: _____ Weight/Reps: _____ Set(s): _____

PRIMAL LIFESTYLE Success score: _____

Item: _____ Comments: _____
Item: _____ Comments: _____

PERSONAL

Comments: _____
_____

One word: _____   Success score: _____

TRAVEL DAILY JOURNAL   DATE: ___ / ___ / ___

1 - 10 SCORE

Energy:	"Big M":	Health:	Mood:	Stress:

DIET Success score: ___

Meals: ___

Comments: ___

EXERCISE Success score: ___   Effort score: ___

Workout: ___

Location: ___   Duration: ___

Exercise 1: ___	Weight/Reps: ___	Set(s): ___
Exercise 2: ___	Weight/Reps: ___	Set(s): ___
Exercise 3: ___	Weight/Reps: ___	Set(s): ___
Exercise 4: ___	Weight/Reps: ___	Set(s): ___

PRIMAL LIFESTYLE Success score: ___

Item: ___   Comments: ___

Item: ___   Comments: ___

PERSONAL

Comments: ___

One word: ___   Success score: ___

TRAVEL DAILY JOURNAL   DATE: ___ / ___ / ___

1 - 10 SCORE

Energy:	"Big M":	Health:	Mood:	Stress:

DIET Success score: ___

Meals: ___

Comments: ___

EXERCISE Success score: ___   Effort score: ___

Workout: ___

Location: ___   Duration: ___

Exercise 1: ___	Weight/Reps: ___	Set(s): ___
Exercise 2: ___	Weight/Reps: ___	Set(s): ___
Exercise 3: ___	Weight/Reps: ___	Set(s): ___
Exercise 4: ___	Weight/Reps: ___	Set(s): ___

PRIMAL LIFESTYLE Success score: ___

Item: ___   Comments: ___

Item: ___   Comments: ___

PERSONAL

Comments: ___

One word: ___   Success score: ___

Cut these pages out for convenient use while traveling.

TRAVEL DAILY JOURNAL   DATE: ____ / ____ / ____

1 - 10 SCORE

Energy:	"Big M":	Health:	Mood:	Stress:

DIET Success score: _____

Meals: _____

_____

_____

Comments: _____

_____

EXERCISE Success score: _____   Effort score: _____

Workout: _____

Location: _____   Duration: _____

Exercise 1: _____   Weight/Reps: _____   Set(s): _____

Exercise 2: _____   Weight/Reps: _____   Set(s): _____

Exercise 3: _____   Weight/Reps: _____   Set(s): _____

Exercise 4: _____   Weight/Reps: _____   Set(s): _____

PRIMAL LIFESTYLE Success score: _____

Item: _____   Comments: _____

Item: _____   Comments: _____

PERSONAL

Comments: _____

_____

One word: _____   Success score: _____

TRAVEL DAILY JOURNAL   DATE: ____ / ____ / ____

1 - 10 SCORE

Energy:	"Big M":	Health:	Mood:	Stress:

DIET Success score: _____

Meals: _____

_____

_____

Comments: _____

_____

EXERCISE Success score: _____   Effort score: _____

Workout: _____

Location: _____   Duration: _____

Exercise 1: _____   Weight/Reps: _____   Set(s): _____

Exercise 2: _____   Weight/Reps: _____   Set(s): _____

Exercise 3: _____   Weight/Reps: _____   Set(s): _____

Exercise 4: _____   Weight/Reps: _____   Set(s): _____

PRIMAL LIFESTYLE Success score: _____

Item: _____   Comments: _____

Item: _____   Comments: _____

PERSONAL

Comments: _____

_____

One word: _____   Success score: _____

TRAVEL DAILY JOURNAL   DATE: ___/___/___

1 - 10 SCORE

Energy:	"Big M™":	Health:	Mood:	Stress:

DIET Success score: _____

Meals: _____

Comments: _____

EXERCISE Success score: _____   Effort score: _____

Workout: _____

Location: _____ Duration: _____

Exercise 1: _____ Weight/Reps: _____ Set(s): _____
Exercise 2: _____ Weight/Reps: _____ Set(s): _____
Exercise 3: _____ Weight/Reps: _____ Set(s): _____
Exercise 4: _____ Weight/Reps: _____ Set(s): _____

PRIMAL LIFESTYLE Success score: _____

Item: _____ Comments: _____
Item: _____ Comments: _____

PERSONAL

Comments: _____

One word: _____ Success score: _____

TRAVEL DAILY JOURNAL   DATE: ___/___/___

1 - 10 SCORE

Energy:	"Big M™":	Health:	Mood:	Stress:

DIET Success score: _____

Meals: _____

Comments: _____

EXERCISE Success score: _____   Effort score: _____

Workout: _____

Location: _____ Duration: _____

Exercise 1: _____ Weight/Reps: _____ Set(s): _____
Exercise 2: _____ Weight/Reps: _____ Set(s): _____
Exercise 3: _____ Weight/Reps: _____ Set(s): _____
Exercise 4: _____ Weight/Reps: _____ Set(s): _____

PRIMAL LIFESTYLE Success score: _____

Item: _____ Comments: _____
Item: _____ Comments: _____

PERSONAL

Comments: _____

One word: _____ Success score: _____

Cut these pages out for convenient use while traveling.

TRAVEL DAILY JOURNAL   DATE: ___ / ___ / ___

1 - 10 SCORE

Energy:	"Big M":	Health:	Mood:	Stress:

DIET Success score: _____

Meals: _____

_____

Comments: _____

_____

EXERCISE Success score: _____   Effort score: _____

Workout: _____

Location: _____   Duration: _____

Exercise 1: _____ Weight/Reps: _____ Set(s): _____

Exercise 2: _____ Weight/Reps: _____ Set(s): _____

Exercise 3: _____ Weight/Reps: _____ Set(s): _____

Exercise 4: _____ Weight/Reps: _____ Set(s): _____

PRIMAL LIFESTYLE Success score: _____

Item: _____ Comments: _____

Item: _____ Comments: _____

PERSONAL

Comments: _____

_____

One word: _____   Success score: _____

TRAVEL DAILY JOURNAL   DATE: ___ / ___ / ___

1 - 10 SCORE

Energy:	"Big M":	Health:	Mood:	Stress:

DIET Success score: _____

Meals: _____

_____

Comments: _____

_____

EXERCISE Success score: _____   Effort score: _____

Workout: _____

Location: _____   Duration: _____

Exercise 1: _____ Weight/Reps: _____ Set(s): _____

Exercise 2: _____ Weight/Reps: _____ Set(s): _____

Exercise 3: _____ Weight/Reps: _____ Set(s): _____

Exercise 4: _____ Weight/Reps: _____ Set(s): _____

PRIMAL LIFESTYLE Success score: _____

Item: _____ Comments: _____

Item: _____ Comments: _____

PERSONAL

Comments: _____

_____

One word: _____   Success score: _____

MACRONUTRIENT VALUES
FOR COMMON MEALS AND SNACKS

FOOD	CARBS	PROTEIN	FAT	TOTAL CALORIES
Broccoli - 1 cup	5.8	2.5	0.3	30
Green olives - 10	1.3	0.35	5.2	50
Brussels sprouts - 1 cup	11.1	4	0.8	57
Apple - 1 med	25	5	0	95
Berries (black, blueberry, raspberry) - 1/2 cup	25	2	1	105
Banana - 1 med	27	1	0	105
Red wine - 5 oz	3.8	0.1	0	123
Hard boiled eggs (2)	1.1	12.6	10.6	155
Dark chocolate - 1 oz	13	2	12	170
Can of sardines	0	22.7	10.5	191
Celery (5 x 4" strips), 2 tbl almond butter	7	7	18	200
Macadamia nuts - 1 oz	3.6	2.2	21.6	203
Venison jerky - 2 oz	8.4	18.3	12.7	225
Beef jerky - 2 oz	6.2	18.8	14.5	232
Sweet potato (1 c with 1 tbl butter)	58	5	12	351
PRIMAL ESSENTIAL MEALS				
Primal Fuel smoothie: *2 c water, 1/2 c ice, 2 scoops chocolate Primal Fuel*	11	20	10	190
Steak and fruit breakfast - *4 oz flank, 1/2 c blueberries, 1/2 peach, 1c green tea*	18	33	10	289
Primal wrap - *salmon, iceberg lettuce, 3 oz salmon, 1/4 avocado, 2 oz cucumber, 1 oz sundried tomato, 2 tbl yogurt*	22	28	13	301
Primal wrap - *chicken or turkey, iceberg lettuce, 3 oz turkey or chicken, 1/4 avocado, 1 oz bacon, 1 oz Bleu cheese, 1/4 c tomato*	11	33	26	411
Primal omelet - *4 eggs, cream, cheese, chopped veggies*	10	27	29	502
Salmon and vegetables - *6 oz wild salmon, 1 c asparagus, 1 c zucchini, 1 tbl butter, red wine*	18	50	26	604
Flank steak and vegetables - *6 oz ribeye, 1/2 c onion, 1 c mushroom, 1 c kale*	21	44	43	639
Beef stir fry - *4 oz beef steak, 2 tbl olive oil, 1 med zucchini, 1 c mushroom, 1 c spinach, 1/2 c bamboo, 1/4 c sesame seeds*	19	41	50	660
Primal salad - *greens, chopped veggies, 3 oz chicken, 1/2 oz walnuts, xv olive/vinegar dressing*	37	24	37	693
Steak and vegetables - *7.5 oz grassfed bison, 1 c spinach, 1 c mushrooms, 1 tbl butter, red wine*	31	70	24	723
Primal Fuel smoothie with coconut milk - *1/2 c coco milk, 1-1/2 c water, 1/2 c ice, 2 scoops chocolate Primal Fuel*	14	22	34	413
***SAD* FOODS**				
Instant oatmeal (1 packet) with medium banana	30	4	2	146
Jamba Juice - medium (Five Fruit Frenzy)	87	2	1	340
Pasta - 1 cup w/ 1/2 c marinana	61	10	5	333
Orange juice - 8 oz	24	2	0	102
Baked potato - 1 med	34	3	0	145
Cheese pizza - 2 slices	30	11	13	279

NOTES

NOTES

NOTES

NOTES

NOTES

NOTES

NOTES

NOTES

NOTES